HAY HOUSE BASICS

ENERGY HEALING

ENERGY HEALING

Unlock Your Potential as a Healer and Bring Healing into Your Everyday Life

ABBY WYNNE

x

HAY HOUSE

Carlsbad, California • New York City • London • Sydney
Johannesburg • Vancouver • Hong Kong • New Delhi

First published and distributed in the United Kingdom by:
Hay House UK Ltd, Astley House, 33 Notting Hill Gate, London W11 3JQ
Tel: +44 (0)20 3675 2450; Fax: +44 (0)20 3675 2451
www.hayhouse.co.uk

Published and distributed in the United States of America by:
Hay House Inc., PO Box 5100, Carlsbad, CA 92018-5100
Tel: (1) 760 431 7695 or (800) 654 5126
Fax: (1) 760 431 6948 or (800) 650 5115
www.hayhouse.com

Published and distributed in Australia by:
Hay House Australia Ltd, 18/36 Ralph St, Alexandria NSW 2015
Tel: (61) 2 9669 4299; Fax: (61) 2 9669 4144
www.hayhouse.com.au

Published and distributed in the Republic of South Africa by:
Hay House SA (Pty) Ltd, PO Box 990, Witkoppen 2068
info@hayhouse.co.za

Published and distributed in India by:
Hay House Publishers India, Muskaan Complex, Plot No.3, B-2,
Vasant Kunj, New Delhi 110 070
Tel: (91) 11 4176 1620; Fax: (91) 11 4176 1630; www.hayhouse.co.in

Distributed in Canada by:
Raincoast Books, 2440 Viking Way, Richmond, B.C. V6V 1N2
Tel: (1) 604 448 7100; Fax: (1) 604 270 7161; www.raincoast.com

A catalogue record for this book is available from the British Library.

ISBN: 978-1-78180-475-9

Interior illustrations © istockphoto.com

Printed and bound in Great Britain by TJ International Ltd, Padstow, Cornwall

*To my family for always being there for me,
even if they didn't know exactly where I was.*

Contents

PART II: THE PRINCIPLES OF ENERGY HEALING

List of exercises

Introduction

I hung up the phone. I knew I had done the right thing. That I had stood up for myself. I was gentle and loving, and he had said sorry, but still I felt the hurt in my chest. I felt the pain in my heart, as if Michael had stuck a knife in, deep in, past the bone and right into the core of me. My ears heard the apology, my brain accepted the apology, but my heart, well, my heart hurt. There was no other way around it. And the hurt stayed there, for hours, days and weeks. And when the sharpness of it eventually wore off, I felt hollow inside, like a part of my heart had died, was switched off, or somehow had left me.'

We have all had experiences where we've been deeply hurt, and usually we understand why. We think about what happened and try to make sense of it. We may even forgive the person for hurting us, but sometimes we still feel the pain even months after the incident occurred. It's as if we are ready to move on in our minds, but some part of us still holds on to the pain and doesn't want to let it go. The pace of our world makes us put that part of us away so we can 'move on' with our lives. When we do that, we often leave

part of ourselves behind, leaving us with emptiness inside. No matter how much we may want to, we cannot think our way out of this type of occurrence.

There is much more to the world than meets the eye. Humans, for example, can't hear dog whistles but we know that dogs can. So logically we understand that sounds exist beyond our hearing range. Similarly, there are colours that our eyes are not able to see, textures so fine we cannot tell them apart and tastes that are way out of range of our taste buds. (Probably just as well!) We understand rationally that our physical body is limited and can only process information within a certain range. Therefore, logically, we can also say there is more information out there than we are able to process. To handle this we label everything, so we can categorize it, and we file it away under 'known' or 'unknown'.

People are also not able to process everything that does fall into our range of perception. There's a famous psychology experiment in which two teams pass a baseball to each other. One team wears white shirts, the other black. You have to count the number of times the white team passes the ball to each other. As you focus and concentrate on the white team, you don't see that a man in a gorilla suit comes in, runs around the players, waves and then leaves. Because you are so focused on counting passes, your brain doesn't notice the gorilla at all. Focused awareness. What you focus on most of the time is what you are aware of. So we actually miss out on a lot of things that are going on!

We can choose what we want to experience, and we can also fine-tune our concentration to block out what we

don't want to experience, just like shutting down that part of us that is in emotional pain. We can block unpleasant feelings or sensations, or the knowingness in ourselves that something is wrong. We learn to ignore things that don't make sense to our brains, like the man inside the gorilla suit, or the pain in our heart that remains months after a break-up.

Sometimes though, we can't ignore these things because they grow too big, too painful. They take over, forcing us to pay them attention. And when we do, that's when the healing begins.

Part I
WHAT IS ENERGY HEALING?

'We are not our bones, we are not our skin, we are the soul that lies within.'
UNKNOWN

Chapter 1
Intuition as a sixth sense

'We were house hunting. We saw so many places! Some of them felt great, but there was one in particular, that felt, well, I don't know how to explain it. Like something bad had happened there. Darkness, nastiness, I didn't understand it. I just knew that I couldn't live there, that something must have happened there that was terrible. I could almost taste it.'

Have you ever had a feeling that something happened in a place before you got there? That the energy of it lingered on long after the incident? Like being invited to your friend's house for dinner, arriving at the door, and even though they greet you with a warm welcome, it feels as if they've just been fighting, and that you have walked into an argument that was quickly ended? Or someone telling you they are feeling 'fine' when you can sense that something is wrong, and they are not fine? This happens when you use your senses to pick up the information behind the scenes, the information that is only accessible by your intuition. As you allow yourself to experience these occurrences, the more

open you become to them and the sharper your intuition will be. As you become more intuitive, you will find yourself 'reading' the information that is all around you, information that cannot be processed by your logical brain.

> *'I was upset to be called in to see my manager. I immediately felt that I had done something wrong, and I became nervous. As it got closer to the time of the meeting, I felt a knot in my stomach, and I began to tremble. I was afraid I was going to get fired. I'm usually afraid I'm going to get fired... Anyway, I went to his office and stood outside the door. I cleared my mind, preparing for whatever I was going to meet. A wave of peace came over me. I suddenly felt that everything was going to be OK. The knot in my stomach loosened. I knocked and entered, and there he was with a big smile on his face, congratulating me for a job well done.'*

When we read information, our brain puts our own explanation on to it, and sometimes we get it wrong. If we have fears or worries, we can put these in the way and miss what is actually going on. Being worried about job security is a fear that some of us hold deeply, and it's very understandable. In the example above, Shirley was connecting with her fears about job security instead of connecting with her intuition. Once she was able to clear her mind of her own thoughts, she could connect with what was really there, which was, in fact, something quite the opposite of what she had imagined.

> *'I was drifting off to sleep, it had been a long day, and I was feeling good. Images of what had happened during*

the day floated through my mind's eye, as I relaxed. Then completely out of context, I saw an image of my dad. I felt like something was wrong, and I woke up with a jolt. I picked up my phone and there was a text from my mum: "Come quickly, dad's not well."'

Sometimes we are like antennae. When we are relaxed and have no agenda for our thoughts we let go of our logical mind, and of our labels, and we tune in to the energies that are around us and experience them for what they are. When this happens, we can learn something we didn't know before we found out about it with our brain.

Maybe you can relate to some of these examples – where things don't make logical sense, but where we get a feeling about something, and we are proven correct even though we do not have a way to explain it. These things happen to everyone, all the time, like knowing your mother is about to phone you before she does, or having a feeling you're going to bump into someone on a particular day, and you do.

We can remain shut down to our intuition, or we can open up and experience the synchronicity of life. We can talk about it, learn about it, work with it and flow with it. This is what Energy Healing is about – acknowledging what is going on right now all around us, inside us and outside of us, even if we don't have a logical explanation for it. Healing is about recognizing what is, and meeting it as it is, instead of using our thoughts to turn it into something else. When we learn to release our thoughts about it and allow ourselves to feel it and accept it, we enable it to move past us, and allow it to change us. We are enriched by the experience of it, and we become better people because of it.

The definition of healing

I have many clients in my healing room opening their sessions with 'This may sound weird but...' and I agree it does sound weird, but the true definition of the word 'weird', is supernatural, not logical. In all of our richness, our beauty, our pain, our madness, we are of the earth and yet we are psychic, multidimensional, multilayered, complex beings of light. You may have felt this. A big expanse of freedom, happiness, light and love, when all in the world is good and everything is beautiful.

Most often though, you have not felt this because we hide our weirdness so that we fit into our culture. We wear a mask, a costume, a smile and go into the world trying to please people; to be good, to work hard, to contribute as is expected of us. We shrink from our full capacity. We disconnect from our weirdness, from our intuition, from our pain and sadly, from our pleasure too. We become less than we actually are, and we go into survival mode.

When I tell my clients that actually it's not weird, crazy or rare but common, and many, many people feel this way, that it's actually very normal, they relax. They feel seen, heard and accepted and gradually safe and able to let go of the mask. They open up and expand, and then they begin to remember who they really are.

Exercise: remembering who you really are

❖ Breathe. Ask yourself this question – who am I?

❖ Close your eyes and focus on your breath, on your breathing.

❖ Feel your body slowing down as you breathe, consciously slow down your breath and become more aware of your body.

❖ You can hear your heartbeat – are you your heartbeat?

❖ What are your thoughts doing?

❖ Can you slow down your mind so that you can be here, with yourself, in the room right now?

❖ Ask yourself – am I my thoughts?

❖ Who am I?

❖ Just be with this question, and if you can, visualize your masks, your protections from life around you.

❖ Are they you?

❖ Do you recognize yourself without them?

❖ Does it feel safe to do this? What would it be like to allow them to fall away?

❖ Breathe. Tell yourself 'It's OK. I am safe.'

❖ Allow yourself to relax a little bit more, every time you breathe.

❖ Repeat this as many times as you need to until you can relax more fully.

❖ Feel your feet on the ground, become aware of the room and then open your eyes.

Healing means being yourself most of the time, not being who you think you should be, or being the person that you think everyone wants you to be. The problem is that being you means that not everyone is going to like you. It means that you might say things that others don't accept, or want to hear. It may mean that you will recognize things in your own life that you don't actually like – things that you have been doing because you feel you should be doing them, instead of because you love to do them. Change will be required when healing takes place, and change is one of the scariest things there is.

Healing means being real to yourself. It means letting go of your masks, your false pretences and the image you put on for the world, and being your true self most of the time. It means you will make mistakes, but hey, you will do that anyway. Life is a learning process, and nobody is perfect. The difference is, when you are healed you take responsibility for your mistakes. You don't go blaming someone else for them, and that's also difficult for most of us much of the time.

Healing means saying 'no' when you need to say no. It means knowing when something is bad for you and respecting yourself enough not to do it, not to go there or not to accept it. Healing means saying 'yes' when you need to say yes, even if you don't want to. It means feeling resistance in your body to something, and knowing that resistance is you saying 'no' because it's easy, not because it's the right thing to do. It means having an awareness of when you are saying no or yes to something, because it is the easy way out. Healing is doing the right thing, no matter how hard it may be, so that you know, deep down

inside, you did the right thing and it doesn't matter who saw you do it. You know you did it, and that is what matters the most.

Healing means forgiving other people, even if they really hurt you, and learning how to accept and bear it, how to face the pain and be with it, instead of running away from it. It means being grateful for what you have, even when you're not feeling it, even when you don't have what you think you should have.

Healing happens all the time, every day, but there is no one day when you wake up healed. It's a process of slowly letting go of what you believe is true, and discovering what is actually true, so you can be real with what is there in front of you. When you are not jumping to conclusions all the time, when you are able to stand back and observe what is going on instead of reacting and taking things personally, you know you are on the healing path.

You can ask for help to heal, you can work on removing any blocks that prevent you from healing, and you can learn how to heal yourself. In your journey of healing, you can also stimulate those around you to heal, but you cannot make someone else heal just because you feel it is what they need.

Healing is letting go of your need to control everything; opening up to the flow of life and trusting that all will be looked after.

Healing is contagious! Just like the flower that grows towards the light, all humans want to move into a state of healing. Give yourself permission!

What is energy?

Electricity is energy. It flows from one point to another, carrying a charge with it, doing work, changing what it touches, bringing light and power from point A to point B. Domestic electricity flows in a circuit that we design, so when you click the light switch, you activate the circuit, the electricity flows to the light bulb and there is light. It's physics! If there is no light switch and no circuit, there is no electricity flow.

We know that electricity without a circuit is dangerous and unpredictable. Lightning can strike at any time, and it doesn't choose where it strikes, it just hits. It can kill trees, people and animals, destroy buildings and cities and cause immense damage. It has no consciousness. It just has light and power.

The information that you 'read' in the background with your intuition, the Life Force that flows through us, is also made of energy. But it is not the same type of energy. We are 'made' of an energy that has a consciousness, a creative energy that can 'choose' which way to flow without a circuit. The laws of physics hold true for this type of energy too. It has a spin, a frequency, a vibration. Heavy attracts heavy and light attracts light but this type of energy is alive. It moves with Divine Grace. It flows from the source of all things, a source of life, Chi, Prana, God, Great Spirit, unconditional love. Because it is outside of our physical bodies' processing range, it is difficult to label. This energy is the energy of our soul.

What is healing energy and how does it work?

Divine Grace, the energy of all living things, has many labels, including: Ki, Chi, Ti, Life Force, Prana, the Body/Mind, to name a few. This essence of grace flows through and around all life forms. Everyone who is alive has access to this Life Force. In the physical body, it flows around organs and tissues and is thought to be responsible for health. As I've already said, our Life Force has a consciousness. So it is connected to our thoughts and our emotions. When we get a shock, or experience trauma or pain, it can block the flow of our Life Force. If we are lethargic or are filling our body with foods/substances that don't agree with us, we may stall or stop the flow. If the flow of this energy is disrupted, the body is affected and can get sick. If the flow stays disrupted, the body can ultimately die. Simply put, Divine Grace, Spiritual Essence or Life Force is what leaves the physical body when someone dies. It's the light behind your eyes.

Exact science to prove that Energy Healing works is difficult to come by because healing is not based on man-made logic. There will always be someone who says it's not real, or that it's a load of rubbish. The difficulty lies with the phenomenon called the placebo effect. When you tell someone that a medicine is going to heal them, and they believe you, then it usually heals them. But what is it that is actually healing them? Is it the medicine, or the belief that the medicine will work? It is difficult to prove which one it is. So if they believe healing will work, and it does work, science says that it's the placebo effect in action.

I want to be completely straight with you. Energy Healing is not an exact science. It is experiential, and you must

experience it before you can feel the effects. You might consider going for an Energy Healing treatment just to find out what it feels like to have one. There is more information about that later in the book, to help you make up your mind.

❖ ❖ ❖

There are two schools of thought around how Energy Healing works.

School one: Energy Healing is a reorganizing of our biological energy field, or 'biofield'. The biofield is made up of the Divine Grace or Life Force Energy that surrounds you as an individual, also known as your aura. When you are healthy, this energy is organized in a healthy way. When you are not, your energy takes any opportunity it can to reorganize itself so that you become well again. Health in this respect refers to your emotional body, your mental body *and* your physical body, as they are all connected and affected by the Life Force Energy.

Reorganization of the biofield can happen through self-healing or by being in contact with a practitioner who has a healthier biofield than their client. The practitioner's biofield acts as a tuning fork, reminding the client's biofield of a better way to organize itself. This is called entrainment, where the stronger force affects the weaker one and brings it up to its level.

School two: Life Force Energy resides outside the body as well as inside it. When it comes from outside the biofield it can be called Universal Life Force Energy, which is available to everyone to draw down from and use for healing purposes. School two says that Energy Healing is the drawing down

of Universal Life Force Energy to replenish and heal an individual's biofield/aura/own Life Force Energy.

When drawn down, Universal Life Force Energy automatically goes to the part of the biofield that is weakest. So we say, 'The energy goes to where it is most needed' as we may not have a logical way to detect this for ourselves.

I believe that both schools are true. I believe that we can do some of the work ourselves using our intention to reorganize our own biofield, and also by giving someone (like a therapist) permission to do it for us. This type of healing can also take place if someone we love has a stronger biofield than we do. It can feel good to hold someone's hand, or cuddle up beside someone who is at peace with the world and themselves. Their biofield can 'tell' ours how to reorganize, and because ours naturally wants to heal, it will respond. Additionally, as the second school of thought suggests, I believe that we can also 'pull down' Universal Life Force Energy, which is a very powerful energy, to help us repair what is broken and heal all the aspects of ourselves.

How can Energy Healing help me?

Energy Healing works at all levels: physical (the body), mental (your thoughts), emotional and spiritual. Because of this, Energy Healing is a very powerful tool that can help you with any issue that may come up in your life. However, when it comes to physical or mental trauma, we may also need to do conventional work to heal the problem fully – if our hip has worn down we may still need to get a hip

replacement. If we have a history of abuse or have been in a war zone, talking to a psychotherapist may be the best chance to help our logical mind.

You can bring Energy Healing into your daily life, but it is not a magic wand to fix everything. You still need to take action to get things done. For instance, if you're looking for a new job, Energy Healing will not get you the job. You will still have to send out your CV and do the interview, but Energy Healing can help keep you remain calm and centred during the entire process!

Using Energy Healing after a break-up

I sat with Cynthia, listening as she told me the story of Michael's betrayal, how he hurt her, how it felt like part of her had died.

She looked at me pleadingly, 'It was two years ago,' she said. 'And I've not had a relationship since. I've been to psychotherapy and I know what happened, but I'm still afraid to let someone else in. It's more than that, it's as if I've got nothing left to give'.

'Are you ready to heal? Does it feel safe now?' I asked her.

'Yes, I'm really ready. I just don't know how to let go of the pain.'

Break-ups are hard, and we take them personally. We mull them over in our heads: where did it go wrong, what did I do, am I a bad person? We can also turn it into a 'blame' game – 'They were so mean to me' or 'They didn't care about me.' Alternatively, we can turn it into a game

of 'What if?' We can easily get caught up in our thoughts and make things worse for ourselves. Thoughts affect our biofield too. The spin and vibration of negative thoughts can bring us right down to sadness, confusion, fear and anxiety. We can almost do more harm to ourselves through our thoughts than was done to us in the first place.

The key to any form of healing is to face the difficult feelings instead of running away from them. You need to be brave to do this. It can be challenging. If it's big, you may need a witness, someone to be there and watch you do this, a friend or a therapist to support you. To hold your hand, so to speak, as you move through your pain. By focusing inwards, doing your inner work, being with the parts that are aching, you heal.

'Breathe, bring your awareness into your body more. Take some time to do this.'

Several minutes pass and I can see from Cynthia's face that she is much more relaxed.

'OK, put your hand on your heart,' I say. 'Tell your heart you're so sorry for the pain, for the hurt that it felt, and that it felt it for so long. Tell your heart that you're here for it.'

She laughs. 'Talk to my heart? Like it's a person? That's crazy!' she says.

'Try it. But mean it – it's about meaning what you say, being real.' I say to her.

She does this, and something in her relaxes at a deeper level.

'Now ask your heart what it needs. What's the first thing that comes to mind?'

'To live again, to have more fun, to laugh, properly, deeply, freely.'

'Do you give yourself permission to live again?' I ask Cynthia.

'Yes', she whispers and tears flow from her eyes, down her face. 'Yes. I do.'

❖ ❖ ❖

Any time you need a space to think, or when you need to bring yourself back to your inner wisdom, your heart or your intuition is when Energy Healing can help. It can remind you not to get caught up in other people's drama. It can calm down your thoughts and dissolve away the details. Energy Healing can help you create new patterns and break out of your old ways of thinking. If you find yourself angry with someone, you can use Energy Healing to relax, release the anger, clear your mind and decide about what to do next, acting out of love instead of reacting out of anger and making things worse.

Remember, the laws of physics hold for the energy of our emotions and thoughts as well as for electricity. When you engage like with like, you amplify. Anger plus anger equals more anger! So if you don't want more anger, you need to bring a new energy in that will dissolve the anger away. Energy Healing! It's not easy to do this at times, as it's difficult to break out of a cycle of anger. This takes time and practice. It's the beginning of life mastery and there

are plenty of exercises throughout this book that can get you started on your healing journey.

Different established Energy Healing modalities

There are many different types of Energy Healing practice, and it can be overwhelming to find one that is the right fit for you. These different types have come about because there are so many kinds of people experiencing the world in different ways. People experience life through their own eyes and work with things that are most familiar – if you grew up around yoga, it would be second nature to you to have a daily yoga practice, but you might never enjoy a martial arts class. So when people try to apply logic to Energy Healing, they put their 'spin' on it and create techniques to go with it. Some people brand, trademark and even 'own' their particular form of healing. That's all fine; there is always more than one way to do anything. However, the important thing for you to know is that the healing energies all come from the same source, no matter what techniques you prefer.

Because there are so many more people accessing healing energies now, there is an abundance of new, and some not so new, modalities out there. (Modality is a way of working).

The most well-known Energy Healing practice in Europe and America is Reiki. You can train in Reiki up to the level of Reiki Master Teacher. Reiki originated in the 1920s in Japan, where you had to train for 11 years before becoming a Reiki Master. When it travelled to America, people couldn't wait that long, so they made it easier. Suddenly, there were more teachers out there, so you can imagine that people started

to modify the practice, and over time, Reiki changed, a bit like Chinese whispers. People began combining other things with Reiki such as crystals, massage, chanting, etc. Reiki has also diversified, and we now have Tera Mai Reiki, Crystal Reiki, Dragon Reiki, Kundalini Reiki; different flavours for different types of people. None of this is a bad thing. In fact, the spreading of healing light across the world is wonderful. However, it is too easy to become Reiki Master now, so it is important for you, as a client, to do your research before you choosing someone to facilitate healing for you. I have included a list of questions to ask therapists in the Resources section (*see page 163*), which I hope will help you to decide who will be a good match for what you need.

There are many purely energetic methods of healing out there, (energy to energy, no diagnosing, no analysing, no advice) such as Johrei, Pranic healing, BioEnergy Healing, Quantum Touch, Restorative Touch, Theta healing, Integrated Energy Therapy (IET), Rahinni, Angelic healing. (For a more comprehensive list see the resources section at the end of the book.) All these modalities have their own techniques that may or may not feel right for you. It's important for you to know that 'no diagnosing, no analysing, no advice' is an ethical standard that most practitioners cannot seem to adhere to, since most clients are very interested in the opinion of the practitioner and are not aware that this is not part of the healing. Please understand that unless a healing practitioner is trained and experienced, has their own healing self-care practice, has done and continues to do their own personal work, and has no invested interest in 'fixing you', their advice may be dangerous if taken to heart.

Some Energy Healing practices are a mixture of talking and energy techniques, in which the therapist is trained in therapeutic dialogue as well as the energy technique, so they may be analysing and working with thought patterns in a structured way. However, taking advice to heart that is outside of the parameters of the therapist's training could be dangerous. You need to be grounded and open minded in any healing session with anyone, and you need to make up your own mind based on what feels right to you.

Types of modality that combine light touch energy therapy with dialogue include Emotional Freedom Technique (EFT), Energy Psychotherapy (where the practitioner is trained in both EFT and Psychotherapy), and Shamanism. I am sure there are many more than this! However, I believe that Shamanism is the basis for all forms of healing, and there are many different forms of Shamanism. Again, you need to do your research into the practitioner and how they work before you go to see them in order to make sure the therapy and the practitioner resonate with you.

Choosing a practitioner

No matter what the modality is, the quality of the Energy Healing that you will experience depends on the person that you choose to connect with. Imagine a coffee percolator. You set up the filter and the coffee and when you put the water in, the coffee comes out. The filter has a certain quality. The coffee also has a quality, and the water is pretty much the same. Apply this to healing. The fabric of the soul of the healer is the filter, the life experience of the healer is the coffee, and the water is the healing energy. Therefore, the quality of the 'coffee' that comes through the filter of that

healer depends on how clear that person is. Unlike actual coffee, we want our healing energy to be as clear and strong as possible. If it comes out weak that may mean that the healers have some work to do on themselves.

Some people are born to be healers. It's in their family, in the very fabric of their essence. They may not even be trained in a specific technique, or they may be trained in several. It doesn't actually matter. Healers of this calibre have a filter that draws down the purest quality healing energy, regardless of how much life experience they may be carrying inside. Just being around these types of healers can create a healing transformation that is powerful and lifelong. At the opposite end of the spectrum, some people will never be great healers because it's not in the fabric of their being. These people have the ability to be great at something else, and the world needs more skills than healing alone! Still, I believe that everyone can heal themselves with a basic framework to work from. Everyone can clear out the 'coffee granules' of their lives and upgrade the quality of their filters. And that includes you!

Even though we are all able to heal ourselves, there are sometimes issues in us that may need a witness in order for them to heal fully. To be in the presence of a healer when you are ready to let go of something can be much more powerful and life changing than doing it yourself. Quantum physics suggests that having an observer changes the state of a process even though we don't fully understand why. I have experienced this with clients who have thought they had let go of something themselves, see it come back up for them in other ways, then come to me to clear it in a deeper way. Don't be afraid to find someone to work with you. If

you have your own permission to do your work, and your intention set to find a practitioner who will help you without doing damage to you, ask the universe to point you in the right direction. Watch the signs that then show up in your life that will guide you in the right direction to move forward.

What to expect during a formal healing session

Each modality will have its own way of being, and the practitioner you choose is best suited to describing what a session with him/her will be like. As for the actual energy transformations in a purely energetic healing session, you may not feel anything at all. Alternatively you may feel some amazing energy shifts, in which your energy moves from, say, heavy and slow dense energies like depression or sadness, into the lighter energy of peace. It really depends on where you are in your life's journey and how much heavy energy you are carrying. It also depends on the fabric of your essence, the timing of the healing, and how willing you are to let go of your emotional pain.

One of the most interesting effects that people report from an Energy Healing session is the sensation of the practitioner touching their head, when they have, in fact, moved on to the feet or another part of the body. Some people fall asleep during a session, and may have lucid dreams or get an answer to a problem that they've been working on. Some people feel as if they leave their body during a session and can see themselves receiving the treatment. Others feel as if they come more deeply into their body. It's a very individual experience, and each time you receive healing, even if it's the same modality and same practitioner, it can be a completely different experience.

I cannot say this enough: the credibility and authenticity of the practitioner are the most important things when choosing who to go to for healing. If you don't feel comfortable or safe with your practitioner the healing will not be as deep, and could even be damaging. Some healing modalities have associations or regulating bodies that create standards and guidelines for its members to follow. In this way, it upgrades the profession and clients have a system of complaint if something should happen in a session. Professional practitioner members of such associations are on a register, and you can go to the website of the regulating body to find one.

Call up the practitioner on the phone and get a feel for them from their voice. Read their website, follow them on Facebook and see if they are coming from the same space as you are. Most of all follow your intuition. If you have a deep desire to see a specific person, that person is very likely to be the one that can help you the most in that moment.

I hope that after you read this book and become more familiar with healing and with your own needs and requirements, you will be confident and secure in yourself and your ability to find a practitioner that you feel comfortable with.

My personal introduction to Energy Healing

When I was in my 20s, I knew I wanted to have children. I had a difficult childhood, and it affected how I saw the world and how I reacted to things. I got angry a lot, and it was difficult for me to control my temper. I knew the type of parent that I would be and felt that was unacceptable. I then

dedicated several years to my own personal development so that I could become the best mother I could be.

I started with self-help books. I read everything I could get my hands on but began to find less and less new information in them that would help me. I wanted to get help from a person too, not just from books, but I had trouble finding a practitioner or a therapy that did it all. Counselling helped, but it didn't change how I felt, just how I thought about things. Hypnotherapy helped me connect with my inner self, but I didn't know what to do once I got in there! Reiki had the biggest impact on me, reducing the intensity of the emotions I carried, relaxing my body and calming my mind. I would 'float' out of a Reiki session and not feel angry, uptight or irritated, which at the time was very unusual for me.

After I discovered Reiki, I would go once a week to see a Reiki Master and have a full hour's treatment, which would carry me through the week. Then life's stresses would build up again and by the time the next week came around, I'd be more than ready for my session. My Reiki Master was also doing a PhD, and over the weeks, she became less and less available to me. Every week became every other week, and it was getting harder and harder for me to hold it all together between the sessions. I realized that I was becoming dependent on her. When she said she was taking a break to focus on her studies, I was thrown completely. I was devastated, in fact. Then she told me that I could learn Reiki for myself. Faced with this reality, it seemed like I had no other choice but to learn it.

After I trained in the first level of Reiki and created my own daily self-practice, I began to stabilize and trust that I would always have it at hand if I needed it. That was very empowering, but it still didn't change how I was thinking about the world and the meaning of life, the universe and everything! I love going deep and picking things apart, learning how they work, so as well as continuing my studies in Reiki, I began a psychotherapy degree. It was great, but it didn't explain how it all fits together, how the very fabric of our being is constructed. At that point, I was better able to handle my anger and the two babies I dreamt about came into my life.

I enjoyed parenting, and I continued to work in my office job at the same time. It was hard. The babies seemed to take everything I had left to give after a day in the office. To keep myself grounded and stable, I needed something that was just for me. I was beginning to understand that spirituality was the bridge between the logical and the energetic. As my questions got more and more complex, I discovered Shamanism, or should I say, Shamanism showed up in my life and scared the daylights out of me!

There are so many mythologies surrounding Shamanism, my fears were around a loss of control of myself, which deeply contrasted with the work I had already put into becoming balanced and stable. Yet there seemed to be something there pulling me in, as if all the answers I had been seeking and more were to be discovered through Shamanism. I had to know more. My babies were now old enough to be left with their dad for a short period of time so I set an intention to go gently, and travelled abroad to begin Shamanic practitioner training.

I continued my psychotherapy degree and held down an office job, now supporting my two babies and my stay-at-home husband. I also managed to travel twice a year to my Shamanic trainings and continued to do deep internal work. I became a Reiki Master Teacher. Just as I was completing my formal trainings two more babies showed up in my life! Four children! For someone who thought they would be the worst mother in the world, I took this as a remarkable gift from the universe and testimony to all the work I had done. I trusted the universe more, and when my work contract was up I had just qualified as a psychotherapist, so instead of looking for another job, I set up my healing practice. What a risk! I was supporting four children and my husband, but it felt like the right thing to do. I was in my power, in my full potential, and the clients came. They sent me their loved ones, talked about the work I did and pretty soon I had a very large network of clients and students. I was very supported. I learned how to blend all the healing modalities together – Energy Healing, psychotherapy and Shamanism to create one seamless, timeless way to heal.

Why I believe you can heal yourself without formal training

Formal training involves explanation of theory, explanation of techniques, and then practice of those techniques. The focus can be more on the techniques than on the healing. 'Do I put this hand there?' 'How long do I stay here?' 'What am I supposed to do next?' That type of thing. Don't get me wrong, formal training is wonderful and important, but you don't need it to heal yourself. With all the new healing modalities, some people have trademarked their

techniques, and everyone says their way is the best way. So there are divided loyalties, and lots of politics. I choose to step away from all of that.

All healing comes from the same source, and the quality of the healer is what makes the healing powerful. And that healer can be you.

My clients come to me in pain. We go on a journey into their pain together, and I teach them how to put the pieces back together, how to heal them. Those that commit to the work continue to heal long after our sessions have ended. Once people know the basic concepts of healing and how to apply them in a practical way, they get better.

They don't teach healing in schools. You've got to start somewhere, so there are some concepts that you do need to learn, and techniques I can give you that will help you experience the concepts in a practical way. Once you have a basic framework for healing, you can go further with it yourself, with or without elaborations, with or without the bells and the whistles.

What I teach I feel doesn't belong to me. I believe that my techniques and exercises come from the source of all things, whether you call it God, the universe, Great Spirit, or unconditional love. I don't want to trademark, register or formalize anything. I most certainly don't want to establish the 'Abby Wynne School of Healing', with accreditations and certifications. What I do want to do is to empower you to understand what healing is about. To show you the concepts and help you experience them. I want to heal the world, by teaching you how to heal yourself.

The only thing I ask is that you keep your work to the highest integrity, that you don't force yourself to do something that you are uncomfortable with, that you don't force healing onto someone who is not ready for it and that you don't set yourself up as a healer after reading this book. This book is really for you alone. If you fall in love with healing while we are on this journey together, then formal practitioner training may be your next step forward.

Remember, only you can do your work, nobody can do it for you. And you cannot do someone else's work for them. So relax, breathe and enjoy the ride!

Chapter 2
Getting started

I have written this book not only as an introduction to the practice of Energy Healing, but also as a way for you to create a path for your own personal healing process.

I want to take you on a journey where you begin to recognize the parts of yourself that you have hidden, and feel safe enough to be with them and tell them that it's all going to be OK. Revealing aspects of yourself that need healing takes courage, and I know and trust that you will look after yourself on this journey and only go as deep as you are able.

With this book, you can make a great start. Bringing your mind, your emotions, your heart, your soul and your body on the journey makes such a difference. If you're reading this book and are seriously thinking about stepping into your own personal healing work, that's wonderful. But if you are afraid of it, if you are feeling the resistance in your body, don't put the book down just yet! Hang in there – feeling resistance to your personal work is a strong indicator that something could change in your life as a result of healing. The resistance is asking you... are you ready?

Exercise: taking time out for healing

❖ Are you ready to heal? Take a minute to think about the differences you will see in your life when healing is happening for you.

❖ Visualize yourself happy, imagine how great things will be and then check in with yourself. Does this feel safe?

❖ Ask, 'What is holding me back from my healing?'

❖ Perhaps you would like to write down your thoughts in a journal. If big issues come up for you, you may need to consider having a witness on your journey of healing. Finding a therapist or a teacher to help you can make life much easier.

I invite you to expect miracles to start coming into your life. Expecting miracles is part of Energy Healing too, and your thoughts around healing are also part of the healing! Energy Healing is not just about putting your hands on your body and thinking yourself better, although that can help. Energy Healing is about reconnecting to your soul, remembering who you are and allowing yourself to be yourself, more of the time.

Be authentic in your work

The key to Energy Healing is authenticity, which means being real or genuine, not being false.

Here's the difficult bit – authenticity means not lying to yourself any more. Not pretending that everything is OK when it isn't, or pretending that things are not OK, when they actually are. You need courage to become an authentic

Energy Healer. You must question what you are saying to yourself. Ask yourself if it's actually true, and have the strength to accept what is true and let go of what is not.

Energy Healing also means being congruent. The healed person knows what their heart feels, understands their gut instinct, and works with both of them. They don't tear themselves apart trying to believe something that they know deep down is a lie.

Congruence: as above, so below

What your brain wants, thinks, or believes is the same as your heart, your intuition and your soul.

So many of us hold ourselves back because we push ourselves too hard in the direction we think we should be going in life, and don't stop to listen to how we feel.

Become congruent

'Every morning I wake with a sense of dread. I don't know what it is; it's like everything slows down. I eat my breakfast slowly and walk to work slowly, like I'm in a movie. Then, as I turn the corner onto the road where my office is, my stomach lurches, like I want to vomit. My heart races, and I think about something else completely. It goes away eventually, usually by the time I am sitting at my desk with my morning tea, going through my emails. But I feel heavy in my body all day, and when it's 4 p.m., it's like the sun comes out from behind the clouds, and I look forward to getting out of there.'

Sandra's job was making her anxious. She kept telling herself that she was suffering from anxiety, to the extent she began to believe she had depression. This is a case of someone telling themselves something that is not real so they don't have to make a change in their lives. Sandra bore the pain of going in to a job that she really did not like, and over time it made her sick.

Being congruent is knowing that your job is making you ill instead of ignoring how you feel and forcing yourself to do what you think you need to do. That is why healing is scary, it may mean that things in your life have to change.

If you're like Sandra and are in a situation that doesn't resonate with you, accepting the way things are instead of pretending everything is OK is actually a better way to handle it. By pretending things were fine Sandra put her mental health at risk to the point where she began to create the symptoms of depression. After a very bad time and several panic attacks, Sandra was forced to look at what was actually going on. She came to me to get some help.

> 'After realizing that it was being in work that was making me anxious I took a week off and rested. It was great to clear my head, do some gardening and visit friends. When my week off was coming to an end, I felt the panic coming back, so I took another week off sick and made this appointment with you. I need the money to pay the bills, I can't quit my job – what do I do?'

> I asked Sandra what she could do to make going into work easier for her while she looked around for another job. She started telling me many things, but they all came from her mind.

'Stop a minute, breathe.' I said. 'Drop down into your heart – what does your heart feel about work?'

'So heavy', she said, 'my heart is so heavy.'

'What images come into your mind with this heaviness? 'I asked her.

'Being at the canteen, people talking, gossiping, stories. Same stories going around and around.'

She breathed with me.

'Now, drop down into your tummy. What does your tummy feel about work?'

'Sick, I feel sick. The people at work are so negative, they're always talking about how bad things are, how awful life is. Being around them, I feel like I've lost hope for humanity.'

After sitting with this, Sandra realized that the actual work she had to do wasn't so bad. It was being around negative people that was making her feel sick. To confirm this, she imagined herself going to work in an empty office, sitting at her desk with nobody around, just doing her work routine undisturbed, then coming home.

'That feels completely different to me', she said. 'I don't feel sick doing the work at all. I actually enjoy what I do. Maybe it's not the work at all that's upsetting me, maybe it's the people in work!'

Isn't it interesting that when you become congruent, authentic with yourself, the real problem can be something that you didn't even realize? Sometimes the obvious thing isn't actually the problem at all! Once you recognize the actual problem, then solutions can appear. Sandra discovered that she was sensitive to energy and was picking up the emotional energies of the people around her. She and I worked on ways she could disconnect from the group energy, release the negativity around her and feel clearer at work, and at home. She began to feel brighter in herself, and could go back to work the following week and feel better about it. Although she found some of her colleagues were not happy with her new way of being, she knew that it was much healthier for her. She eventually did get a new job just to change her environment, and was able to recognize negative group energies and not get involved with them. The exercises that I used with Sandra are in this book, so if this story resonates with you, you're in the right place!

How to use the exercises in this book

Please bring your whole heart and soul into your healing practice. And your brain too! Be authentic. Be congruent with yourself. You have to allow yourself to feel the exercises, to be open to them, for them to change you. This is when the magic happens. If you hide things from your Self you will have trouble doing the work.

You may be a beginner at Energy Healing, but you're not necessarily a beginner at life. The richness of your life experiences makes you who you are, and that counts. There is no right or wrong when it comes to these exercises, so you cannot compare your experience of healing to someone

else's. It's like comparing your Chapter 1 to someone else's Chapter 16! They have their work to do, only they can do it, and the same goes for you.

Each exercise is designed to be repeated many times. So if you're having trouble with one of them, do as much as you can do, then leave it and come back to it another time. But do stick with it, be patient with any resistance you may be feeling, as each time you do the exercise you will break through a little deeper. Know that resistance to some of these exercises could be you just getting ready to let something go and move to the next level. A little bit of resistance is natural and good. However, a strong resistance towards one of the exercises may mean that you're not ready for it yet, so don't push hard, wait until you feel ready.

These exercises have to be heartfelt to be useful to you. You can go through the motions, say the words and not feel anything at all, and then tick the box that you've done them. But you haven't, not really. I would rather you stick with one exercise until you feel you've got it working for you, instead of racing through the book and trying everything half-heartedly. Allow the information and the healing to seep through you, like the warmth of a long, hot bath. You have plenty of time to do this work. You've got the rest of your life.

Remember, healing is about feeling better, being confident, happy and well. Clearing what is in the way of being well through these exercises takes time, patience and dedication. When you feel the results of the work you put in, there's nothing like it! It frees you. The relief is indescribable,

suddenly there's magic and colour in the world. You have to experience it to believe it. Words don't do it justice. You'll enjoy the feeling so much you'll never want to go back. You deserve it (yes, you do!) and if you keep up your practice, you can feel that way most of the time. Energy Healing is a practice. Remember, you're never finished healing.

If you do not feel the energy shifting in your body when you try the exercises, I would suggest that you persist with them regardless. It's possible that you may need to break through some sort of energetic wall or blockage before you really begin to feel the changes.

I have had clients that have never 'felt' the energy, but they've seen it or have just known that it has moved. And if, after trying for a long time, you still don't feel a result, you could consider booking a session with a healer to see if they can help you move through whatever is blocking you from moving forward. Again, there is information about how to find a therapist in the Resources section *(see page 163)*.

The mechanics of Energy Healing

Our vibration

Imagine a guitar string: when you pluck it, it vibrates. The speed of the vibration is the frequency, which is the note that you hear. A low vibration would give a low note, and a higher vibration would give a higher note. You can feel vibrations in your throat when you sing, low vibrations on the low notes, high vibrations on the high notes. We have a vibration too – our Life Force Energy vibrates. As we

experience life, learn things, are influenced, our vibration changes, or shifts. As we experience emotional pain, trauma and distress, our vibration gets lower. When we experience joy, happiness and peace, our vibration gets higher.

Holding on to pain shuts off the flow of energy through our body. Blocking our natural flow affects our vibration by lowering it, and if we don't process and let go of our emotional pain, the blockages can also cause physical pain. If not attended to the physical pain can cause mechanical damage, chemical damage and affect our metabolism. You can visit a physiotherapist for a frozen shoulder, get your exercises and lift weights to get stronger, but if you don't deal with the emotional pain you are feeling, the energies may stay blocked and your shoulder could always be a problem for you in your life.

Energy Healing goes straight into the energy system of the body, relaxing and releasing the blocks, opening up the flow and raising its vibration. By working directly with the energy and releasing the blockages you get the benefit of the physical pain lifting, and then the body can heal itself.

Emotions have a vibration

We all have days when we feel heavy and slow, like we can't get out of bed; these are when we resonate with heavy and slow vibrations. Our vibration affects our choices and our moods, so on a low-vibration day we may choose to listen to sad music, wear dark colours, eat comfort food and not want to spend time with people. We also have days when we leap out of bed full of the joys of living and make high and fast vibrational choices including wearing bright

colours, listening to upbeat music, eating healthy foods and being sociable. We have more energy when we are at a high vibration, and we have hope and motivation. We feel productive and creative.

Energy Healing works directly with the vibration, not with the emotion, so you don't need to name what is going on. Our brain, however, does like to know what is going on, so when you recognize that you feel sad and your brain wants to know why, that's OK. But if you're working with a vibration of a sadness that's been in your body for a long time, it might not be as helpful to try to make sense of it. Sometimes you have to step away from the brain, from the needing to know, and just accept that you're feeling sadness. What can help when this happens is to remember that the feelings are a vibration that you are experiencing in that moment, they will pass, and you are still you regardless!

Shifting low-vibrational emotions

When you practice Energy Healing you may 'pull down' a high-vibrational energy into your body. Due to the laws of physics, low-vibrational energies cannot stay in the same place as the higher ones – if you have a darkened room, and you turn on the light, it's not dark any more. You don't get an 'instant hit of happy' with Energy Healing because it's rather like a drip feed, slow and steady, and you have to come into balance with the energies and stabilize. But you will feel more grounded, more relaxed and more like yourself again. Know that we are not our sadness, just because we feel sadness. Remembering this when you feel down, and using Energy Healing to feel better is very

empowering and much healthier than spending your time analysing why you are sad and not shifting the vibration.

Over time, with a regular healing practice, your body will carry higher vibrational energy for longer amounts of time. This means it is possible for you to feel good more often than you feel bad. Feeling good can become the daily normal for you, and you will only feel bad if there is something wrong.

Be patient with your healing practice

Imagine a swimming pool, beautiful, fresh and clean. Then someone goes and throws a bucket of dye into it! If you are not allowed to drain the pool and start again, the only way you can remove the dye is by flushing it out. You attach a pipe to one end of the swimming pool for the new water to go in, and a pipe to the other end for the old water to go out. Let's say you turn the tap on and the new water pours into the pool, and the old water starts to flush out. The first few hours of doing this, it won't look like anything is happening at all. Even if you leave the tap on overnight, the pool would still have dye in it the next day, but you might begin to see an improvement. After another 24 hours, you could probably see the bottom of the pool, and perhaps by the third day, the water would be clear enough to swim in.

So when you 'turn on the tap' on you, with your Energy Healing practice, the new high-vibrational energy flows into you, and then the old stuff that you don't want gets shaken up, shifts and leaves. The amount of 'dye' in your 'swimming pool' is based on your life experiences and your

ability to process them and let go. This is why you cannot compare your results with healing to anyone else's. Some of your old, heavy vibrational energies may take years to shift, particularly if they are blocked in your physical body, but sometimes the old, heavy energies are ready to release, and leave really fast! If you're congruent, you can say goodbye to your pain and let it go much more easily than if you're incongruent and are trying to let go of pain that you're not actually ready to let go of yet.

Why people don't heal

One of the reasons people don't heal is incongruence. Hiding something from yourself because you are not able to accept it, or don't want to work with it, is a form of denial. Your body knows it's there, your soul knows, but by your brain consciously pushing it away and acting as if it doesn't exist, you become incongruent. Incongruence is a big block to healing and this is why I'm spending so much time talking about it here. If this is something that you think you are doing, that's great, because now you can stop doing it! Be gentle with yourself, you're not doing anything wrong. This is a natural thing. You might want to take some time to nurture yourself, give yourself permission to look at what might be in the way of you becoming congruent on your healing journey.

There are a few other reasons why people don't heal – you can't let go of emotional pain that you're not ready to let go of yet. Awareness and being gentle with yourself really help here; understanding the source of the pain that you struggle with can help you do whatever you may need to do, before you can let it go.

Consider Mary, whose grandmother had passed away. Mary had always loved her grandmother's opal ring, and when everyone was in the house for the funeral, she went up to her grandmother's room and took it from the jewellery box. She didn't tell anyone, and when her grandmother's things were being gifted to the family, they noticed the ring was missing. Mary didn't speak out about what she had done, and was too afraid to wear the ring, as everyone would know she had taken it.

Mary came to me because she had started seeing her grandmother everywhere. She felt haunted by her image and was anxious, stressed and upset. Mary wanted to heal, and we worked together, but it seemed to get worse for her. She couldn't forgive herself for what she had done, and because of this, she couldn't grieve for her grandmother. She had to tell her mother that she had taken the ring. Her mother understood and forgave her and then Mary was able to forgive herself. That's when the healing happened.

Grieving is a necessary process when we experience loss in our lives. It enables us to let go of emotional pain around the loss and come into balance with our new life situation. Mary actually had to take action and speak to her family before her consciousness would allow her grieving process to take place. Gaining forgiveness for what she had done was the permission she needed to allow herself to heal.

What is blocking your healing process?

Is there an action you need to take in order to clear anything in you that is blocking your healing process? Take some time now to open up gently and reveal to yourself anything

you may be hiding from yourself. You don't have to share this information with anyone, but you do need to become aware of it.

The main reason why people don't heal is the fear of who they will be when they are healed. As Marianne Williamson says, 'We are more afraid of our light, than of our dark.' It's as if we believe that once we are healed we will have to be perfect and aren't allowed to make any mistakes, and we can no longer blame anyone else or have any excuses for our failings. This is not true. As a healed person you are still a human being, and as a healed person you will still have your lessons, your mistakes and your learning to experience. Our learning continues until the day we die; there are still plenty of new experiences to be had to enrich our lives. I will talk more about this in Chapter 7. Just know at this point, if you have trouble feeling like you deserve to be happy and pain-free and to have a good life, then you might need to consider doing work to increase your self-worth and self-esteem.

Don't give up on yourself, no matter what you discover. All things will unfold as they should, and if you make a commitment to heal (and follow through on your commitment), then you will heal, perhaps not as quickly as you would like, but you will heal, I promise.

❖ ❖ ❖

The power of intention

Intention is a decision to do something. It's an aim, a plan or a direction. Intention is usually set within the context of what you want to do with your day, or with your life

– 'Today I am going to have a good day', or 'He studied medicine with the intention of getting a job as a doctor.'

Intention is fundamental to healing work. You need to set an intention to heal before the healing will happen. A healing intention must be in alignment with all the aspects of yourself, all the aspects of your soul. (Alignment meaning on the same side, and in agreement with.) So, if your intention is to go to college and study medicine to be a doctor, but your heart wants you to be an artist, you're not in alignment with your decision.

That's a big example – but again, if you're not ready to heal something and your brain is pushing you to 'get over yourself and heal it' like Mary was, this creates more resistance. Then the healing becomes more painful than it needs to be. Healing is an organic process – it's natural, and only happens when you are ready. The first part of being ready is to set your intention to heal.

Exercise: setting your intention

❖ What would your intention have been when you bought this book? Can you put it into one sentence? Say it out loud now and see how it sounds.

❖ Has your intention changed since reading the first two chapters? What do you think has brought about the change?

❖ Awareness is key to your healing. Recognize that your intention needs to be aligned with your mind, your heart and your soul. Breathe, and voice your intention to heal.

❖ Breathe, make sure your two feet are on the ground and place your hands on your stomach. Does it feel tight or soft? Does it flutter with anxiety, or is it stable and in balance?

❖ Say your intention out loud again and see if it helps relax you a little more deeply.

❖ Know that you will feel better as a result of a daily healing practice.

The power of permission

Yes I know it sounds funny, but sometimes you get so used to feeling bad you're afraid to feel better. Permission is very powerful, and if you don't give yourself permission to heal, you won't accept the healing. Permission is also important when you are 'sending' healing to someone else, and we will talk about that later, but it is important for you to give yourself permission too. It's like opening a door and sometimes, when you set the intention and give permission to heal, that's actually all that it takes for the healing to happen. Very powerful!

You can say it out loud, or you can say it quietly to yourself, but it's best when you quiet your mind and focus your awareness on what you are doing and feeling. Try to bring your mind into the present moment and don't get caught up in thoughts around how, why, when or anything else.

Exercise: learning to give permission

Here are some different ways to give permission; try them out and see which one fits you today. Remember that tomorrow you will feel differently and you may need to choose a different one.

❖   I give permission for healing to happen.

❖   I give my full permission to heal.

❖   I open my heart and let go of anything in the way of my healing.

Notice if you feel anxious when you say this; you may need to relax, breathe and say it again. Do you mean it 100 per cent? Really?

If you don't that's OK, ask yourself why, and come back and try again later on.

The power of receiving

You've set an intention and now you've given permission. See how it's all building up! Now you need to open and receive.

How do you know if you're really opening up to receive? Imagine you've bought some new clothes, and your friend says 'I love that outfit on you, you look amazing!' You say, 'Not really, it's just some new clothes...' and brush it away. That's not receiving what they're saying. Your self-esteem and self-worth have an influence over this. If you have low self-esteem, it's harder to accept a compliment.

Let's try again. They say how amazing you look and you say, 'Thank you!', and you blush and turn away, and close down your heart because it's not really possible that you

would look amazing. Well, it's better, but you're still not receiving the compliment.

Let's try one more time. They say how amazing you look. You look them in the eye and you stay there. You don't run away in your mind, but this time you feel it. Imagine that the compliment they sent you is a ball of light, coming from them to you. You stay and accept it. You feel a shock or a hit from the light as it enters and becomes absorbed into your system. Like a shiver! Then you say, 'Thank you, I appreciate you saying that.' A higher vibrational energy (the compliment) coming into your system can feel strange, even painful, in a good way, depending on what vibration you are carrying in that moment. That's why we run from compliments; they change our vibration, if we let them.

Now you know how to receive properly. Try this exercise for real the next time someone says something nice to you. Then you can say something nice back to them in return.

Exercise: opening to receive Energy Healing

Soften your resistance to healing by imagining a door in your mind that now opens to let the healing come in. Remember the swimming pool? Well, if your water is warm and the new water is cold, you will get a shock from the temperature change. So let's imagine the Energy Healing is the same temperature as you are, so that it feels gentle and good, so that there are no shocks involved. You could also imagine you're opening both of your hands to receive a gift, or you could imagine a box that was buried deep in your soul, one that has been closed for years, is being dusted off, and now is ready to open to the light. See it open in your mind. 'Yes! I am ready.'

❖ Sit comfortably where you won't be disturbed. Set your intention for healing (a simple 'I want to feel better' is a good intention).

❖ Give your permission to receive. ('I give myself permission to receive healing now and feel better'). You can say this out loud, or in your mind.

❖ Now, allow your imagination to use one of the images I gave you above, or to create your own image of how you open and receive. Just doing this is like a green light for your biofield to reorganize itself, so you might notice some energy shifts even at this point. Take some time and let it happen, slow down and notice if you feel uncomfortable, joyful, if you receive an energy burst, or have a breakthrough with an issue that's been on your mind.

❖ If you feel uncomfortable, become aware of what you are thinking about – I don't deserve this? I'm not good enough? I feel guilty for receiving this gift?

❖ Healing is a gift, and there is no need to feel guilty, because it is your birthright. You'd let a stranger receive the light, why not you? Be nicer to yourself, tell yourself it's OK, and stay with this exercise. Repeat it over a few days until you feel more comfortable with it.

Healing can get worse before it gets better

So now you know that Energy Healing is not just about healing with energy. It's about being true to yourself, not running away from your pain, releasing old wounds and changing your life.

Healing *can* get worse before it gets better – have you ever given up sugar or caffeine? There's a detox period in which your body releases the bad chemicals that were bound up in your body, and you can feel ill from that. You can have a terrible headache, you can be dopey in your mind, need to sleep or just feel rotten overall. But if you persist, after a few days your body clears, and then you really start to feel the benefits. You may feel lighter, more awake and have more energy. The same thing can happen with healing. It's called a Healing Crisis, but it won't last, and when it's done you will feel much better. So, don't give up!

Going into process

Swimming pools catch leaves, sticks, even bits of stones and gravel. Imagine as the new water goes in to clear the dye, it stirs up the pool a little and the debris floating on top gets forced into the out pipe, and then blocks it. More water forces it to move, but it is blocked and slow. Once the debris is eventually pushed through to the other end, it comes out with a 'POP!' and it's gone. The pipe is clear again and the pool is that bit cleaner, but the process wasn't easy. Imagine how much water is needed to force the debris out of the pipe.

When you start a healing practice, you go 'into process', which means the waters in your 'swimming pool' get all stirred up and then start to flow in the general direction of being clear. You're much more complex than a swimming pool, but if you were one, you might have gravel, leaves and mud, but you might also have bits of broken cars, shopping trolleys, even glass, depending on what you have experienced in your life. When you start healing you don't

know what dirt is going to get churned up, what bits of sticks and debris may end up blocking your pipe, so to speak.

Look after yourself during healing

I want you to be aware of this so that you can be your own watchdog and make sure that you look after you. Sometimes you might be healing for days and not feel any result, like you're pushing the water into the pipe, and the gravel isn't moving. You might even feel physically ill or emotionally upset, and not know exactly why. Memories of things that you've forgotten about can surface, and you may find yourself trying to make sense of what's going on for you. Don't. Just know that you are in the process of healing, and that these stuck energies are moving, and will eventually leave, so that you can be at a higher vibration than you were.

You don't have to do this alone. If you want to get help don't be afraid to ask. Talk to a friend, to someone in your family, or find a practitioner to help you, if it's too difficult to do it alone. Check out the Resources section (*see page 163*) and you can always ask me questions by email or visit me on my Facebook page.

Part II

THE PRINCIPLES OF ENERGY HEALING

'Healing is a different type of pain. It's the pain of becoming aware of the power of one's strength and weakness, of one's capacity to love or do damage to oneself and to others, and of how the most challenging person to control in life is ultimately yourself.'

CAROLINE MYSS

Chapter 3
Centring

Many of us think our way through life. We use our brain to navigate everything: where we are going, what we want to eat, what we choose to wear. We even decide how we feel. We live in an intellectual world surrounded by things to stimulate our minds, and if we don't have a project, a hobby or a problem to work through, our brain goes back to our past, or flies into our future and 'chooses' something from there for us to become preoccupied with.

When we tend to be in our heads most of the time, it's as if our Life Force Energy follows, moving up to be more in our head as well, because that's where we're focusing our attention. Sometimes our Life Force Energy moves up and out of our head, and outside our body too.

Think about it – have you ever felt like you haven't fully arrived somewhere yet? Or notice that when you drift off into your thoughts, you lose connection with your body? How about right now – do you feel that you are fully present in your physical body? Do you know what your feet are doing? Do you know what your legs are doing? Now

that you're thinking about it, did you notice a shift in the energies of your body? Are you more aware now of your feet? Start to notice how much you drift, and know that your Life Force Energy also drifts with you.

Let's get started with some basic Energy Healing exercises!

Creating a space of love

To begin your healing practice you will need to create what I call a space of love for yourself. Some people call this a sacred space, but love is sacred, so it's the same thing. A space of love is a quiet space where you feel completely safe, and will be undisturbed. You can go all out and burn a candle or incense, play soft quiet music, dim the lights. But you don't have to do any of that if you don't want to. Feeling safe in your space of love is the most important thing.

It's best to treat all these Energy Healing exercises as work and to be wide awake for them so you can experience them to the full. Sit up straight with your feet on the ground, or sit on the ground if you prefer. However, if you want to use any of the exercises in this book to help you fall asleep, your intention will then be to fall asleep, rather than to do healing work. You can go ahead and do them lying down, but make sure that you also do the exercises while awake so you don't just sleep through them all!

You can set a space of time around your exercises too if you want to, it's completely up to you. Time can help you feel secure in your space of love as well. If 15 minutes feels too long, try 10, and remember that even three minutes is better than no minutes! If you choose to set a time boundary around an exercise, know that sometimes doing

that can help you go deeper into it. It's as if you give your mind permission to concentrate fully on the work at hand as it will only be for a set amount of time. Wonderfully, sometimes after an exercise things don't seem as urgent or as important as they did before, so this helps with stress management too! If you set an alarm, make sure you use a soft tone so that you don't get a shock from a harsh buzzer breaking into your relaxed state.

Your space of love can be used as a setting for all the exercises you do from the book, or for any type of ongoing healing practice that you may choose to create for yourself. You can set a space of love just to experience the different energy you feel while inside it.

Exercise: being in a space of love

❖ Take some time to create your space of love. Set your alarm if you wish to set a time boundary.

❖ Set an intention to sit in the space of love just to be with yourself, just as you are.

❖ Sit for as long as you feel comfortable and breathe, relax and let your mind wander, not having to do anything, just being present to whatever is going on for you.

❖ Don't get caught up in thoughts. If you do, just disconnect and bring yourself back to your breathing, back to being in the space.

❖ Notice how you feel – do you feel different now?

❖ Come back to yourself. Feel your feet on the ground, and bring your awareness back to the room.

What was that like? Was it difficult just to be still or was it easy? Do you feel refreshed? Calmer? Or more agitated? What would you like to change about your space of love, if anything?

Notice that this is your starting point, before we get deeper into the healing work. If you were feeling nerves, agitation, anything like that, it's OK. It's natural. In your normal daily life do you tend to avoid quiet, peaceful times? Do you always have to listen to the radio or television, or be on the phone or on Facebook? Try this exercise again with a time boundary, or without one if you used one already, and notice if it feels different to you. Just learn, there is no right or wrong, there just is what there is. We start from this place.

Reconnecting to your body

'I don't feel happy or joyous. It's been about five years since I really felt alive. I want that feeling back. I need something to change but I don't know how to do it.' Tucking a loose strand of hair behind her ear, Carol looks distant and sad.

'When was the last time you felt connected to your body?' I ask. 'I mean, really in your body, fully present, here and now?'

'Hmmm... I don't actually remember.'

'Let's start by introducing you back to your body, saying hello to it, no pressure to do anything, no pressure to be anything – would that be OK?'

*She sits up in her chair, but moving slightly back and
away from me. 'I'm not sure – what does that mean
exactly?'*

*'Well, your body feels, that's its job. You think thoughts,
but your body feels the emotions that go with them
and only by processing the thought and emotion
together can you truly embody change. I suppose the
main problem is if you've not felt anything in a while,
you can become afraid of what it is you may feel when
you come back to the body experience. It's perfectly
safe – you don't have to do it all today.'*

'Maybe. I'll think about it,' she says.

❖ ❖ ❖

It can be difficult to reconnect with your body if you have
been away from it for a while, so here I suggest a very
gentle exercise, coming back into your body and saying
hello, as if it's an old friend whom you have not seen in
a long while. Doing this might bring up difficult feelings
that you may have for your body; you may not be happy
with parts of your body, or you may feel discomfort being
in your body owing to physical pain. Becoming centred in
your body is very important though, because it's only here,
in your body, that you can access your full potential.

You can do this exercise in segments over a longer period if
it becomes overwhelming, or you can take some time to go
deeply into it. If you feel anxious just thinking about doing this,
take out your journal and check in with yourself. Ask yourself
why you feel anxious. What's going on for you? Go outside
for a walk, clear your head, then come back and try again.

Exercise: becoming centred in your body

❖ Sit comfortably in your space of love. Have an open posture, no folded arms or crossed legs. Close your eyes. Bring your awareness to yourself, to where you are focusing your attention right now.

❖ Breathe.

❖ Imagine that your attention, your focus of awareness, is a ball of light. It is usually outside your body, so if you locate it outside your body, that's perfectly OK!

❖ Give yourself a minute to settle with this, and you may notice that as you pay more attention to this centre of awareness, the ball of light in your mind's eye may get brighter and stronger! Just let it be whatever it is.

❖ Gather up all of this light that is you, outside your body, and invite it to come and sit at the top of your head, over your crown. Notice as you do this you may feel a shift in your energy.

❖ Imagine this ball of light has moved up and is now directly over your head, shining brightly there, bringing you more awareness of your actual head!

❖ Breathe, and allow yourself to settle like this for a moment, and give thanks to your energy for taking part in this exercise.

❖ Now with your next breath, invite this ball of light to come gently through your skull, and into your head. Don't worry, it won't hurt. Feel it dropping in, and imagine the light shining from the inside of your head, out through your eyes, washing your brain clear of negativity, opening up your ears.

❖ How do you feel doing this? Breathe, and keep your focus and awareness on your head, on the light inside your head. As it shines

more brightly, you relax more deeply with every breath. Go slowly, feel every bit of this if you can.

❖ You're still not centred right now. You're in your head! Better than being outside it. Does it feel different to you? You can stop here if you want to and come back and try again another time.

❖ Breathe. On your next out breath, imagine your centre of awareness, your ball of light, dropping down into your mouth. Feel it shining out from behind your teeth. Bring your awareness more deeply into your mouth, your tongue and your cheeks. Stay in your mouth for as long as you feel comfortable; imagine that you open your mouth and the light shines out. Imagine this light is cleansing and purifying the cells in your mouth, tongue, cheeks and even your teeth.

❖ Breathe softly and deeply. Allow your centre of awareness, the beautiful ball of light, to drop down gently into your throat. Notice if your throat tightens up as you do this, and tell yourself 'it's OK'. Breathe with the light, and notice if you relax, or if you don't. Feel your attention and awareness still with your throat, then bring it to the back of your throat, to your neck, and imagine the light is feeding the cells in your throat and neck and they're getting a 'drink' of healing from you.

❖ Breathe again, and feel your feet on the ground, bring your awareness to your throat again and now allow the ball of light to drop down into your chest. Become aware of your shoulder blades, the tops of your arms. Notice how you feel, how your chest feels – is it tight? If it is tight, stay with it and breathe a little bit longer, give yourself permission to relax, and enjoy this sensation of being in your chest.

❖ If it helps, you can imagine that you have armour around your chest, and each time you breathe, the light that you are shining melts the armour, and you feel more free and open. If this feels scary to

you that's OK too; perhaps this virtual armour is a shield you are carrying as protection from the outside world. Remind yourself that you are in a space of love, and you are safe. See if that helps. Again, you can stop here if you don't want to do any more, and come back later and try again.

❖ Breathe, and allow the light to drop down to the centre of your chest, to your breastbone. This is your heart centre. Breathe, and imagine the light inside you lighting up your rib cage, breathe big and strong and then relax the breath, soften and notice how you feel.

❖ Normally, when at the heart centre of the body, people feel more centred. How do you feel now? Maybe write it down. I see the whole body as the centre, the sky as the above, and the ground as the below. So for me, centring isn't truly complete until you are in your whole body.

Ready to keep going?

❖ Breathe and get your bearings. Make sure that you're actually still at your heart centre. There could be a tendency for you to shift back upwards as you become more familiar with the feeling. If so, bring yourself gently back down again, and you'll notice that the more often you do this, the easier and the quicker it gets.

❖ Drop your focus of awareness, your ball of light, downwards to just above your bellybutton. Use your breath to do this as before. This is the part of the body that most people are very conscious of; they hold that belly in tight!!

❖ Remember that you're in your safe space now, you may need to tell yourself that it's all OK, and that you're fine just as you are in this moment. Again, you might have trouble believing that, but do your best to relax with yourself, with your body. You can change anything if you really want to; perhaps getting to know yourself at this deeper,

physical level, will help you make some changes too, if that's what you want to do.

❖ Soften and relax your stomach, let it all hang out! Nobody's looking!!

❖ When you're ready, imagine the ball of light, the centre of your focus and awareness, dropping down to just below your bellybutton. This is where many people hold the most anxiety, so go gently here, feel your feet on the ground, and breathe with yourself. Slow down if you need to. Bring your awareness into your belly, into your lower back, into your spine. Just feel what you feel, and know that it's all OK. Again, you can stop if you want to and come back later for more.

❖ Breathe, and drop down into your pelvis. Imagine the ball of light splits into two parts, each part moving into one of your hips. You have two smaller balls of light, one in each hip now, shining brightly; you might become more aware of the chair you are sitting in when you do this. Let these balls of light gently and slowly move down your legs at the same time, moving into your thighs and down to your knees. Imagine the balls of light now moving from your knees, down the front of your legs, together and at the same time, into your ankles and then into your feet. Imagine your foot bones lighting up, touching the floor.

❖ Breathe. You are centred in your body now.

'How do you feel now?' I ask Carol, after doing the body reconnection exercise with her.

'Different. Not really sure... heavier, but much more peaceful.'

'It's funny how we're not allowed to feel heavy, as if being heavy is something bad. It's not bad, it's how it feels to be in our body, until you get used to it!'

'Yes, that's what it is,' says Carol with a smile. 'I'm in my body! Wow!'

Being centred in your body is a great place to be when you have to make decisions, think clearly or be present for other people. If this is the first time you've felt like you've been in your body in a long while, I recommend you try this exercise every day for a few days to settle into it before continuing with the rest of the work in this chapter. And if it takes you a few tries to complete the whole exercise in one go, that's wonderful work, well done!

Notice what brings you right back up and out of your body again! A loud noise outside? Or a thought? Maybe you could check in with yourself at different times of day, notice where your focus of awareness is and pull it back into your body. It gets easier the more you do it. You will find that after a while, doing this becomes second nature to you, and that you have more awareness, and are more able to be present in the moment. It's a gift!

Listening for a 'yes' or a 'no'

When you connect to your centre, you have access to your intuition. Your intuition is part of the very fabric of your being, your soul essence, the Life Force Energy that makes you, you. Images are the way that our soul speaks to us. The soul has no language; words are something that our minds created. For everyone, the experience of communicating with his or her intuition is different. Some people see an actual image before their eyes, some get a taste in their mouth, a shiver down their spine, or hear an inner voice, while others experience a sudden knowingness.

You probably already know how your inner wisdom reveals itself to you, but you may also be an expert at avoiding listening to it.

Our brain is impatient and likes to jump in and guess before we actually get a chance to really connect. This is something you need to unlearn. Before you can truly believe that the wisdom you get from your intuition is a real message from your Self and not just something you've made up in your head, you need to know what a 'yes' and a 'no' feel like. Are you ready to do this? Be as real with yourself as you can, as this will aid your authenticity and integrity in your healing work.

Exercise: listening for a 'yes' or a 'no' (intuition reconnection)

❖ Create your space of love, with the intention to feel a 'yes' and a 'no'.

❖ Sit, breathe and relax. If you need to, come more into your body using the centring exercise, until you feel as if you've arrived.

❖ Work on a yes first. Tell your body you want to hear/feel/know a yes.

❖ Ask a question to which you know the answer is yes, such as 'Is my name...'? 'Do I live at...'? Ask if your family are your family. If your favourite book is the one you love best. Ask as many times as you need to in order to feel the yes, learn the yes, resonate with it, recognize it.

❖ Then work on the no. Ask yourself something that you know is a no, such as 'Am I SCUBA diving right now?' Think of as many questions as you can where the answer is obviously a no and ask yourself those – notice how the no feels different in your stomach, in your chest.

❖ Now breathe and centre, letting go of the thoughts. This is clearing a space, like cleansing your palate at dinner. Now say out loud 'yes yes yes yes yes' and notice how that feels, if it maps to what you were feeling earlier. Let the wave of 'yes' shift away from you, come back to centre. Now try with a 'no no no no no', and again, map that, anchor the feeling into yourself so you will recognize it later.

❖ Now really use your intuition by asking a question that you don't know the answer to. Not a serious question, but one you are interested in knowing the answer to, such as 'Am I making all this stuff up?' or 'Am I feeling OK right now?' Wait and feel your body's response, your heart's response, your gut's response. Is the yes and no response clearer now?

❖ Don't pressure yourself for an answer, your system is only getting used to having your full attention and it might jam up! It might also jam up if you ask the most serious questions first, like 'Am I on track with my life?' or 'Should I leave my job?' Give yourself time to grow into this, practising it with any choice you need to make, or any question you know has a yes or no answer. Confidence using this yes/no intuition exercise will come over time, as you get the results you expect.

Connecting to your heart

Your heart is the seat of your emotions. On a good day, your heart centre shines its light to the world, radiating love. On a not-so-good day your heart centre can shut down and hide from the world, hoping nobody sees it. We can very quickly disconnect from our heart centre, and get back up into our heads, into our minds, thinking about how we should feel, telling ourselves how we do feel, without actually knowing how we really feel. And if something should hurt or upset

us it's very easy to shut our heart centre down, although not so easy to wake it up again.

> *Cynthia's boyfriend Michael betrayed her, but even after forgiving him her heart shut down, and months later, when she thought she was ready to move on with her life, her heart still felt the pain.*

> *'It's like I feel dead inside sometimes, like the colours have drained out from the world. Nothing seems to bring me joy. I'm with a crowd of friends, they're laughing, and I'm laughing too. But I'm not really laughing, not laughing on the inside. I don't remember the last time I really felt happy.'*

Having a closed heart can make you feel disconnected from life. Energy Healing can help awaken your heart, help you feel more connected and bring the colours back into your day. But you have to feel safe. It comes back to being authentic, being congruent. If you have a closed heart because of years of abuse, you have to make sure you've worked through the issues in your mind that stop you moving forward. Energy Healing can still help soften the mind, soften the emotions, but it can be a long process.

Now we are going to reconnect with the heart. If you get caught up in your thinking, you are getting distracted from the work. Ask yourself if what you see/hear/imagine is real, wait for your yes or your no. If it's a yes, keep going. If it's a no, regroup, centre yourself and start again. This takes practice.

Our brain has a lot to tell us, and we do need to pay equal attention to the mind, the heart and the soul. Nobody gets

left behind! Reassure yourself that you will listen to all of it, but this time, it's your heart's turn to speak to you.

Exercise: connecting with your heart centre

❖ Create your space of love and make sure you feel safe.

❖ Set your intention to reconnect with your heart, to be gentle with yourself.

❖ Give yourself permission to go as deeply as you feel comfortable, and to stop if you need to.

❖ Sit with open body posture, check in with yourself and ask yourself if you are feeling nervous about doing this. If you feel nerves or tightness in your stomach, tell yourself it's OK. Go at your own pace.

❖ Imagine your focus of awareness, the ball of light, just as before. Bring it into your body, just like before. Take as long as you need to, and you can stop when you reach your heart centre.

❖ Breathe and feel your feet on the ground. If you are feeling light-headed at this point, continue with the exercise like before, bringing the ball of light down into your pelvis, down into your legs and into your feet. Then bring your awareness back up into your heart.

❖ When you feel connected to your heart centre, breathe and relax even more deeply. Open up your chest. Imagine the armour or protection you carry around you is melting away.

❖ Now step into your imagination and visualize a garden. It could be one that you have visited or seen before, or it could just be one that materializes in front of your mind's eye. It's a beautiful garden, and at the back of the garden is a flower; this is the flower of your heart.

❖ Move towards the flower as if it is an emotional being and you don't want to frighten it. Notice what type of flower it is, and whether the petals are open or closed. Ask permission to sit, and then when you feel it's OK, imagine that you sit down beside the flower. Look at it with kind eyes, appreciating the things that this flower has been through, the pain and the trauma, the fear and the anxiety. You are a bringer of hope, you bring with you love, and healing. Ask the flower if it's OK to heal now, and see if it feels right. Breathe, and imagine that this flower is breathing with you, in and out, in and out.

❖ As you're breathing in and out, both of you breathing together, you can visualize a glow of healing light coming down from the sky, through the top of your head, down through your body and outwards from your heart centre. This healing light is silvery gold. It's beautiful high-vibrational energy and feels like champagne bubbles. It flows around you, through you and across to the flower. Helping you both to soften, relax and heal.

❖ On the out breath, all the stress and tension you're both carrying flows to the ground. On the in breath, new, fresh energies come in and feed your soul. And you're looking at the flower, and the flower is looking at you, and you're breathing together. Your heart is opening, along with the flower.

❖ If there are any blemishes, tears or sore patches on the petals of the flower, see them healing and repairing themselves with the healing light. If the stem looks stark, visualize the healing light feeding your flower and the stem thickening up, fresh new leaves growing on it.

❖ Ask the flower what it needs from you. Does it need some quiet time to rest? Is there anything you can do in the physical world, the day-to-day life, that would help your heart feel better? Wait and listen.

❖ Now, give thanks. Visualize the healing light dissolving away gently, leaving you both revitalized and glowing. It's almost as if you bow to the flower, and the flower bows back to you. It's time to go. Put your hand on your heart and imagine yourself standing up to leave the garden. Tell the flower you'll come back and visit again, and visualize yourself leaving the garden; as you do this, come back into your body gently, and back into the room, into your space of love.

❖ Take a moment or two to reorient yourself. Notice how you are feeling. You might want to write down what comes to mind, what the flower said. You might want to draw a picture of your flower, or find a picture of it on the Internet and use it on your phone as a screensaver to remind you that your heart does have the capacity to open.

If your heart flower opened only a little bit, healed only a little bit, it's a great result. If your heart flower acknowledged your presence and breathed with you, that's also a wonderful thing. And if all that happened was that you got into the garden and saw there was a flower there, then that's also wonderful. Even if you got to the garden and there was no flower, that's still a good first step. Come back again tomorrow and wait, the flower may be too upset to show its face just yet. Trust me, we have very high expectations, and that can be the pressure that breaks the healing process. Step back from what you expect, and be with what actually is.

By your showing up, your heart learns to trust that you do actually care, and it shows you a little bit more of itself every time.

Tuning in and disconnecting from the energy around you

As you get more familiar with yourself, with your intuition and your heart, you will notice all of the things that affect it that you may not have been aware of before. Remember Sandra with her job? She realized that connecting into heavy, slow, group energies was making her sick. You may also begin to realize that the group energy you are exposed to has the same effect on you.

This next exercise is one you can do when you are surrounded by other people, and find yourself caught up in their emotions. This is difficult to do if you have not spent time centring yourself in your own space of love, so if this exercise appeals to you, make sure you spend lots of time learning how to get centred when you're on your own first.

You can use visualizations to speak to your soul, to give it an instruction, depending on your intention. So in the case where there are people around that are upsetting you, you can visualize a bubble surrounding you, disconnecting you from their emotional energies, and lifting your vibration. By being strong in the visualization you're actually telling your soul you want to disconnect from the other people, and it will listen to you and do it! It's remarkable.

You don't actually create a real bubble around you. What happens is that you reorganize your biofield energetically, pull your energy in and become more consolidated, and at the same time you push out the energy you don't want and that helps you feel stronger.

Your bubble can shift and change in your mind's eye – the colours and the texture of the bubble can be different depending on the situation, your imagination, or the energies that are involved. Let it be what it is without trying to influence it, it could surprise you! It might not even be a bubble at all – I have a client who told me he imagines himself as a tank when he walks down dark alleyways, a big strong tank with armour and a gun facing outwards. He said that it makes him feel much stronger and safer, and that nobody ever approaches him when he does that.

You can do this exercise quietly while still paying attention to what is going on around you, and the great thing about this is nobody will know you're doing it. It's very empowering to be able to push away the heavy energies that upset you. It helps you get your focus and take your power back from a situation.

This next exercise takes it one step further; try it and see how it feels. You can then choose to do the short exercise when you feel you need to and the longer one (below) when you're at home and you have more time.

Exercise: creating a power bubble of protection

❖ Set your intention to create a disconnection between you and any heavy energies around you that are not yours.

❖ Locate your centre of focus and awareness. If you have trouble doing this just ask your Life Force Energy to come back to the centre of focus and awareness (try it – it really works!).

❖ Using your intention, draw the centre of focus and awareness closer to your physical body and feel your energy coming back to you from the others in the room. You can draw it into your heart, your head, your stomach, wherever feels appropriate to you at that time. (Like a quick version of centring – but this is by no means a way to do the other exercise quickly! It's more like an emergency response.)

❖ Visualize a bubble around you, 365 degrees. Even if people are standing close to you, that's OK, your bubble is energetic. They may even feel it and move a little further away from you.

❖ Make sure the bubble in your mind's eye is strong and clear, so you can see out of it, breathe inside it and see that there are no tears in it. Check the quality and strength of the bubble, particularly behind your back, too, as we tend not to check there so much.

❖ Now breathe, and feel your feet on the ground. As you breathe, imagine you're pushing any energy that is not yours outside the boundary of the bubble. It might take a few breaths to feel like you've really cleared a space for yourself. You might find yourself getting light-headed, so place your feet on the ground and slow down the breathing.

❖ Notice how you feel. Now if you think the bubble is too small, breathe and use your imagination to tell your Life Force Energy, your soul, to expand the size of your bubble until you feel more comfortable.

❖ Over time, the bubble will dissolve away as you will lose your awareness of it, and your energy will mix and match with that of the environment again. You need to be constantly centring yourself and putting energy into making the bubble for it to be active. As you do your healing work you will expand naturally by yourself, and you will notice that you don't need to create a bubble of protection around you any more.

Centring is very important to learn, and once you have worked with all the exercises in this chapter and are comfortable doing them, you can move onto the next principle of Energy Healing: Grounding.

Don't be afraid to come back and revisit these exercises if you need to – all these aspects of healing go hand in hand and it's important to get them all working together.

Chapter 4
Grounding

If someone was described to you as 'really grounded' or 'down-to-earth' it might bring to mind images of someone who is realistic, calm, centred and authentic. Do you know anyone like this? What are the qualities in them that you resonate with? Is it an attitude or a way of being? What does being grounded mean to you?

I want you to think about this, because the conventional idea of 'being grounded' and the energetic 'being grounded' are two different things altogether.

When you have your feet on the ground, a clear head and don't get carried away by intense emotions, you could be said to be a grounded person. Some people choose certain activities to help them feel grounded, such as yoga, art classes or walking barefoot. None of those actually grounds you energetically unless you bring your intention to do just that. Most people are not aware of this, so they'll say they feel 'really grounded' after doing those activities, but they're not energetically grounded. Most of them are just more present in their body.

In energy work, grounding means much more than being present in your body. In fact, energetically you could be a down-to-earth, grounded person, when you're simply centred most of the time!

Imagine a tree. It reaches its branches up to the sky to get to the light, but if it is windy and the tree has no roots, it will fall over. The taller the tree is, the harder the fall. It needs an anchor, something to attach it to the earth, so that it can be strong, steadfast and ride the storm.

If you're not confident with the exercises on centring in the previous chapter, you might need to take some more time with them before you start the work here. You need to be energetically centred in your body before you can go more deeply into the ground.

Why do we need to ground ourselves?

People who are ungrounded can feel unbalanced, uncentred, scattered or even confused. I find that making my best decisions happens when I am grounded in my body because this state of being helps me connect to my inner wisdom. Many of my clients experience panic or anxiety because they are not grounded in their body; it's their body panicking because they are not connected to their source of power, their source of wisdom, it's as if they're out there in the world with no protection, no resources to draw on.

'It can strike me when I least expect it. I feel hot, that's usually the first sign, and then I know the panic is coming – my mind starts racing... Once my mind starts it's like

I can't stop it. My thoughts push me over the edge. It doesn't matter if I'm alone, or surrounded by people – my stomach feels like there are a thousand trapped butterflies trying to escape, I want to vomit. My breathing is so fast and my head starts to spin and I become very unsteady, I have to hold on to something. When it's really bad I completely forget where I am, I lose focus, I can't see, can't hear... During those times I feel like I am watching myself having a panic attack, like I'm not really here experiencing it at all. I want someone to come and take me away, to lock me up. Sometimes I want to die just to make it stop.'

This description is from one of my clients describing a full-blown panic attack, which is a very scary thing to experience. You can also have anxiety attacks that are not as violent, or have a low-level, constant feeling of fear or anxiety from not being grounded in your body. It really does help to be grounded. I have seen so many people's lives transform because they have a daily practice of centring and grounding themselves. Suddenly, the world feels like a safer place. They can go to the shops or meet friends and not worry about the possibility of having a panic attack. It's remarkable how this simple piece of energetic work can result in transforming a life so dramatically.

Grounding is as if you are throwing an anchor from your Life Force Energy into the earth that holds you down strongly and keeps you secure and safe so you can go about your life. The difference between feeling held and feeling like you're floating away is the difference between a calm and stable physical body and one that panics because it feels

alone. Maybe this is a simplistic way to see it, but I believe that our bodies are an aspect of us that love us and need love from us in return. Once we are in our body, it feels loved and it does its best to love us back.

Exercise: grounding yourself with the help of a tree

You can do this outside with an actual tree, or you can do it in your mind's eye with a tree that you know from home, from a park, or one that you visited a long time ago. If you try this the first time with a real tree, you can then call on your tree in your mind anytime you need help when you're out and about doing other things, and need to ground yourself quickly.

❖ Set your intention to ground. You must be centred first, so check in and notice where you are in yourself.

❖ Breathe, catch hold of the focus of your awareness in your mind, and bring it softly down through your body, starting at the top of your head then all the way down your spine, into your pelvis, going down each leg, strengthening each leg and opening the energy flow of your body. See your hips in balance and your legs strong. Don't do this quickly so you become fully centred in your physical body.

❖ Go to your tree – either in real life, or in your mind. The tree is bigger than you; walk right up to the trunk of the tree and connect in with it – touch it, say hello with your energy to its energy. Notice how tall the tree is, how the trunk rises high above you, how the branches and leaves reach right up to the sky.

❖ Ask the tree if you can work with it. (It's always polite to ask!)

❖ Imagine your energy is now merging with the tree, stretching up high with the branches, but also moving down, down deep to the root system.

❖ In your mind, imagine yourself travelling down through the ground, the mud, the stone, with the tree, to the deepest, longest strongest roots. How does this feel?

❖ Now you can imagine your energy wrapping itself around the root of the tree, so it can hold you deep down below the earth. Bring your focus of awareness back up to your body, leaving your energy down there, breathing out any fear, anxiety or heaviness you may be carrying. Feel your feet on the ground, feel yourself in your body fully, feel strong and tall and long like the tree.

❖ Say thank you to the tree! Then you can either let the image dissolve away, or you can walk away, and you are grounded.

Deeper grounding

Set some time aside and use grounding as the intention for an Energy Healing meditation. This is very helpful if you are feeling low-level anxiety on a constant basis. It gives you and your body a break from it. Be completely real with yourself, taking a few minutes before you start to check in and ask what's going on for you. Sometimes changes in life or conflict/confrontation with a loved one can unground you, and no matter how grounded you may feel after a meditation, something that's important can quickly undo the good work you've done. If you need to take action, make a list of what you need to do. Don't be afraid to ask for help.

Exercise: achieving deeper grounding

❖ Sit in your space of love and set your intention for a healing, deeper grounding practice.

❖ Connect into your focus of awareness. Draw it down your body slowly, with each breath. Take a good few minutes to do this, dropping down softly and slowly, opening up your body and relaxing more and more deeply with each breath.

❖ Bring your awareness into each part of your body, dropping down into your pelvis, your hips, down your legs, your knees, your calves, your ankles and your feet. You may even want to travel down your arms, your elbows, your wrists and your hands too. Feel your body's Life Force Energy flowing through you. Visualize all your energetic blocks melting away, your body coming to a deep state of relaxation.

❖ Feel your feet on the ground. Bring your focus of awareness completely to your feet. Imagine your foot bones lighting up, going into your toes, spreading out and connecting you to the earth.

❖ Move your focus of awareness to beneath your feet, then to the skin on the soles of your feet. Imagine you can feel each cell in the sole of your foot touching your sock or your shoe, and breathe.

❖ Now imagine your focus of awareness is going down even more deeply – through the floor, the ground, into whatever is next. Do this slowly, too, imagining what it is like inside each layer, what each texture breathes like, smells like, tastes like... If it's dense or humid or heavy, or light and spacious. If you are inside a building, then imagine you are moving down through the building: the steel framework, the foundations, down down down deep until you hit the soil underneath. Then go into the soil, deep down into the nurturing, richness of the layers where the roots of trees and plants live.

❖ Stay here for a moment and feel the shift in your energy, feel the heaviness, the comfort, the holding from the earth. Relax and be comfortable here, feel the love that Mother Earth has for you. Breathe and relax.

❖ Imagine that there is a sweet spot in the earth that is pulsating with Mother Earth energy. Tap into that in your mind and then breathe into it, connect with it then breathe it up, breathe up the energy of earth, a soft, red mist, a loving, nurturing warm energy. Breathe it up through the energy connection you created when you were going down. Breathe it right up through the building if appropriate, and up into your feet, keep going! Breathe this energy right up into your stomach.

❖ Now you are connected to Mother Earth energies, and you are connected to your own flowing Life Force Energy. Use the breath to do a cleansing.

❖ Breathe out the fear, the anxiety and any heaviness you are carrying, right into the earth. Imagine it is going down to Mother Earth, she's taking it from you, to recycle it, to feed the flowers, to purify the soil.

❖ Breathe up the energy from the earth, up into your legs, your legs getting stronger, more open, breathe it right up into your stomach and feel its peace, its strength, its beauty.

❖ Do this breathing four or five times. Deep breath up from the earth and hold. Deep breath out and let go. Deep breath up from the earth and hold. Then deep breath out again, and let go.

❖ Relax. Let go of the breath and just sit, feel the energies mixing in you.

❖ When you are ready, slowly bring your awareness into the room. Dissolve away any images that you've created and allow your energies to settle. How do you feel?

What did you feel when you did that exercise? What did you notice in yourself? Were you comfortable doing it? It's interesting when people do this exercise and bring their full attention to it because they notice things like one leg is easier to work with than the other, or that they feel more in one side of their body than the other. It's all OK, there is no wrong or right, there just is what there is in this moment, right now.

If you're feeling your energetic blocks strongly, it could be because it's been a long time since you were in your body, and your body may be having trouble accepting you. Your body also carries memories and trauma from your life that your mind may think you've already dealt with. Parts of your body can shut down because your focus of awareness has not been there for so long, as you are unconsciously (or sometimes consciously) avoiding the memories, and the emotional pain that you experienced.

Remember, Energy Healing is clearing the emotional energy, but sometimes you do need to work with the memories that are still stored in the body, too. Bringing your brain in helps you to change your perspective, to forgive and to let go of emotional pain. Don't be afraid to get help, to find a witness, to heal. It's the best thing you can do for yourself and the best thing you can do for the world.

Why do we go down when we ground?

One of my clients refused to go down when we did grounding in a session. She was Catholic and deeply religious, and became scared in case she was going down to hell. I want to be clear – grounding is nothing to do with religion. In

fact, energy work is nothing to do with religion. Energy Healing is empowering, active spiritual work. Because it is empowering, because you connect directly to the ground, (and in the next chapter you will be connecting directly to the sky), there is no interpreter of what is happening for you. There is no priest or church needed for you to have direct connection to the Divine Source, Energy of Grace, to Universal Life Force, Healing Energy, or Mother Earth. You don't have to turn Pagan, run rituals under the full moon or join a religious group. Neither should you feel you should leave a group to which you already belong. This is spiritual, not religious. Spiritual is about your connection to yourself, to the universe. Spirituality is where there are no rules, only experiences, and they all come from a place of love.

I believe that we can live in heaven or hell right here, right now, in our physical bodies, on this planet. We don't have to wait until we die. We can be outside ourselves, ungrounded, disconnected from our intuition, navigating life completely from the mind, suspicious of everyone, afraid of competition, jealous, angry and holding on to grudges and emotional pain that make us sick. Or we can be connected to our hearts and our intuition, let go of our pain, be responsible for our behaviour and our choices, and use our minds as a tool for kindness and healing. We can be living in the worst life of our imaginings, but we can turn it around and start to create our best life. Most of us are living in between the worst and the best, but we can make choices to move into the best without feeling guilty for doing so. We are here to shine our light, so the first step is to allow ourselves to do just that.

Shall we continue?

Quick ways to ground yourself

Sometimes you need a quick grounding fix when you're out and about, and the simple technique with the tree is a great one to call on if you've already put the time in and are familiar with the process. If you're feeling really ungrounded and wobbly and need something even quicker, you can imagine you're pulling energetic roots up out of the ground (a bit like jack in the beanstalk tendrils). See yourself wrapping these energetic roots around your feet to hold you to the ground.

You can also imagine putting on shoes that are made of lead, or that your feet are sinking through the floor, or that you are connected to the energy system of Earth and you just need to plug yourself in. You could see yourself throwing out a rope from your body with a big anchor on it, the anchor going through the ground and into the earth. Or you could imagine spikes or corkscrews growing down out of your feet and into the ground. All of these images are instructions from you. You are telling your Life Force Energy what to do, and it does just that.

As time passes and we get absorbed with other things, we may slip out of our grounded state. Notice when you feel ungrounded, and ground yourself again.

Grounding when you're in the air!

You can actually ground yourself wherever you are, even if you're in a plane or on the top of a Ferris wheel! Of course, if you suffer from vertigo, this might not be enough. Don't feel as if you're invincible once you can ground yourself, as there may still be other things that you need to attend to.

Exercise: grounding with the Earth

❖ Imagine yourself standing in a field – your whole body and with your feet on the grass.

❖ Imagine yourself growing very big; if it was a cartoon, it would be like your body growing bigger and bigger, as if you were becoming as big as the city you are in, the street you are in, the country you are in, with Earth staying the same size.

❖ Zoom out of planet Earth, see yourself growing bigger and bigger still, so that it looks like you are standing on top of the whole planet now, and the planet looks small beneath your feet.

❖ Now imagine you are dropping an anchor from your pelvis, or from your stomach if you really feel ungrounded, right into the centre of the Earth.

❖ Feel the tug, the pull, when the anchor connects to the Earth's core. Feel your feet flat on planet Earth and know that you're grounded.

Grounding in the crystal cave in the centre of the Earth

These exercises use a lot of imagination, and remember what you are doing is using these images to tell your energy what you want it to do. And it's doing it! Even though your physical body is still in the room where you left it, your energies really are travelling around the place and reorganizing.

When we go deep into the ground in our imagination, we leave a part of our Life Force Energy down there with the roots of the trees. But that's good, as it holds us, connects

us to this planet that we are living on, and then we won't feel a need to connect to someone or something else to feel secure.

In this exercise, we will go more deeply into the Earth – right into the Earth's core where we will find a crystal cave. All of this is magical and imagination play, yes, but it allows for deeper grounding energetically, and you will *feel* the difference in you, rather than trying to *analyse* the logic of it.

So, let go of what is real in the physical world and come on a journey with me into the metaphysical, where we will ground deep down into the Earth's core.

Exercise: grounding in the crystal cave

❖ Create your space of love and make sure you are comfortable. Your intention is to relax and ground your energies in a deep way.

❖ Bring your focus of awareness to the top of your head. Ask for all your Life Force Energy to participate in this exercise. (You can say it out loud – 'I ask that all of my energies come into the room right now!')

❖ Notice how you feel after doing that. Breathe, and relax your body.

❖ When you are ready, drop down into your body, slowly, breathing the focus of your awareness all the way into your head, your neck, your spine, vertebrae by vertebrae until you reach your heart.

❖ Stay at the heart, open your chest and breathe out any emotional pain that may be in the way of you doing this exercise. Take as long as it takes to move through it.

❖ Breathe, drop down to your stomach, relax your stomach and breathe out any emotional pain, fear or anxiety that may be in the way of you doing this exercise.

❖ Take as long as you need until you feel you are fully present in your stomach.

❖ Drop down again, this time into your pelvis, down your legs, knees, lower legs, ankles and feet.

❖ Just as before, imagine that your focus of awareness is dropping through the floor, through the building if appropriate, and into the earth below.

❖ Drop your imagination down past the roots of trees, down, down down, right to the Earth's crust. (Sometimes I imagine dinosaur skeletons here!)

❖ Keep going through the mantle of the Earth, into the Earth's core, where the fires burn and the molten lava moves like a red-hot sea. The lava and the fires feel cool although they look red-hot, they burn away heavy energies in your energy body.

❖ If you want to stay here for a while you can imagine you are giving anything that's holding you back to the fires of the Earth to be burned away. This can be very healing, so if something has come up for you during this chapter around trauma or emotional pain, use this opportunity to see yourself pulling the energies out of your body, saying goodbye to them and throwing them into the fire. See the fire burn them away.

❖ When you feel ready, imagine you see a small cave. You walk into it, and look around; take sometime to adjust to the energies here. At the back of the cave is an even smaller cave, which seems to glitter and call to you, so you move towards it.

❖ Inside the mouth of the cave is the biggest quartz crystal you have ever seen, several times bigger than your physical body. Imagine you step into it and are absorbed by it. You can feel the quartz energies healing you, purifying you, raising your energetic vibration. Stay here as long as you like.

❖ When you're ready, step out of the crystal, and into the cave itself. At the back of the cave are many more crystals. Choose one that calls to you. You can pick it up, turn it over, and look at it in your hand. Notice the colour, the texture and the clarity.

❖ Place it somewhere in your body. Remember it's your energetic body you are working with so you can gently place the crystal into your legs, your pelvis area or your stomach. Feel the connection between that crystal and the other crystals in the cave, as if they are glittering or pulsing together.

❖ You can spend some time here exploring further, or you can get into the giant quartz crystal again if you want to.

❖ When you're ready to return to your physical body, give thanks to the room, to the caves, and come out back to the centre of the Earth.

❖ Step through the fires, and let them wash you clean. Leave behind any energies you are not supposed to bring back with you to your physical reality.

❖ Now imagine you are moving up, up through the crust of the Earth, back the way you came, following the same path, seeing the same things, back and back, up up up to the building you are in, to the room you are in. Breathe gently as you enter your physical room. Breathe and enter your physical body, feeling grounded, solid and strong.

❖ Take your time to stretch, open your eyes and bring your awareness fully back into the room.

You can have some fun with this exercise if you want to. Allow it to evolve as you change over time. While you are in the cave you can wrap your energy around the giant quartz crystal and use it to ground you, or you can leave something in the cave that weighs you down, and let the fires burn it when you are not there. You can even go back to the smaller cave on another occasion and swap the first crystal for another one. All of this work is happening not in this reality, but in the energetic reality. Real healing is going on at a level of your energy that you don't logically understand, but you can feel it in the flow of your Life Force Energy, you can feel it in your body, you will notice it as you feel more self-confident and strong.

Grounding when you're distressed, over-emotional or panicked

Here's a quick way to ground yourself and release strong emotions at the same time. This is great when you are feeling overwhelmed, which can happen from time to time as you release old, stagnant energies during your healing practice. Hopefully you will never need to use this, but it's always good to know just in case. If you can do this outside on the grass, near a tree, it can be a very powerful exercise.

Exercise: heart-to-Earth grounding

❖ Clear a space for yourself and lie face down on the floor, grass or ground.

❖ Breathe and allow the emotion to come up in you; it's safe to cry if you need to.

❖ Feel your heart opening with the ground beneath you, a direct connection to Mother Earth.

❖ Imagine energy cords connecting from your heart straight into the ground, and from your pelvis straight into the ground, holding you fast and strong.

❖ Feel secure and know you are held by the Earth.

❖ Imagine a trapdoor opening in your heart and a second one opening in your stomach. Allow the heavy emotional energies just to fall right out of you; dump them like you were a rubbish bin dumping the contents into a landfill.

❖ Wait until you feel emptied out, and then use your breath to steady yourself, and to keep you in your body.

❖ If there are tears, allow them to flow. If you do cry, become soft in your tears and come back to yourself slowly.

❖ Feel your body, feel the floor beneath you.

❖ Let go of the images, come back and notice the sounds around you. Notice the temperature of the air on your face. Notice your breath. Wait until you feel steady before you get up.

❖ Have some water, a cup of tea, or a gentle walk to help settle you back into yourself.

Always look after yourself when you are in the process of healing. Take some time to ask yourself what you need to do to help yourself feel better. And do it!

Grounding yourself to shift a bad attitude

We pick up on the energies around us and can tap into the energy of our community. The media likes us to buy into the worst possible scenario and we may be carrying weight in our energy system from the news reports we watch or listen to. When you wake up on a Monday morning do you feel like you have the troubles of the world on your shoulders, or do you leap out of bed looking forward to the day? People tend to hold on to the bad stuff for longer, so dreading the week ahead is actually trained thinking. We are built to survive, there is a programme running in our heads that keeps us focused on possible threats to our safety. That may seem fair enough, but some of these 'threats' are ones we make up ourselves, and are not real. Do you ever find yourself thinking, 'It's going to be a terrible day today' without even really asking yourself if that is true or why you feel that way? We tend to think of the worst possible scenario more often than best possible scenario (trained thinking again), and we feed each other the worst possible scenario too. When you're constantly on high alert, you create a stress hormone, your stomach suffers and you disconnect from your body, becoming ungrounded.

When we get upset, frustrated or anxious, the tendency is to go up into our thoughts, out of our body. When we are anxious, we feel it in our stomach – it tightens up, it may feel like butterflies, or churning, even nausea. This is most unpleasant. I'm sure you've experienced one or all of these sensations. The first reaction we usually have when we feel anxiety is to disconnect from sensation, and we quickly move up into our thoughts to avoid feeling ill, but by doing this we disconnect from our intuition, and that's

what we need to be connected to at times like this, to handle whatever the situation may be.

Usually when fear resides in our stomach, it's about not feeling confident or safe. Sometimes we create the feeling of insecurity by thinking things about a situation that are not true. The biggest fear that some of my clients have is a fear of having a panic attack. This fear of having a panic attack is fear that is manufactured. They create it themselves, and if they didn't, well, it wouldn't exist. So when we create fear-based thoughts, we then feel anxious or panicked, and we create more fear-based thoughts, thus the cycle keeps us feeling stressed, out of our bodies, away from our intuition and up in our heads.

We can always change our attitude, even if we cannot change a situation. What if you could change your attitude towards something that stresses you, right now? Being grounded helps you see through the fears, helps you get connected to what is real and disconnect from what is not real, so you can let go of the fear and come at the day with a much healthier attitude.

In this exercise, we mindfully set an intention for the day, breathe out the fear, ground ourselves, and feel more secure and much less stressed.

Exercise: grounding intention for the mornings

❖ Catch your thought process and swing it around. Instead of thinking, 'I hate Mondays and, even worse, today is a rainy Monday,' you could think, 'It's Monday. It's raining, but I'm alive, I can hear my breath. I am grateful for this day.'

❖ Now breathe, feel your feet on the ground and let go of your thoughts.

❖ Breathe, and come into your body, centre and ground through the floor and into the earth. (Take as long as you need to do this thoroughly.)

❖ Now set your attitude. 'I will make the best of today. Just as many good things can happen as difficult things. I open my heart to notice the good things more than the bad.'

❖ Give yourself permission to step into a vibration of lightness, of ease, of calm and of peace.

❖ Breathe out anything that is not peace, calm or lightness.

❖ Believe that you can achieve everything you need to do this day. You could even say out loud 'I can and I will!'

❖ Now isn't that better? What else could you apply this grounded thinking to? See if you can shift other attitudes you have, using this way of thinking.

Grounding yourself for better decision-making

I remember the first time I went into a grocery store in America. It was many years ago, and at that time in Ireland we only had a few supermarkets to shop in; there was not

much choice of food available either. For bread, you could choose brown or white. For biscuits or cookies, you could have chocolate-covered or plain. I was overwhelmed by all the choices in America, not just for bread and biscuits, but for restaurants, clothes, music... I went into a record store and my head was spinning. What did I choose? Nothing. I couldn't choose. There was too much to choose from. It felt better to walk away. I was overwhelmed.

There are so many choices for everything right now. How do you know what is the best choice for you? Some people I know can't even decide on a movie to watch or a book to read, let alone what to study or which career path is for them. Being overwhelmed by choice can knock you out of your body. Conscious grounding brings you back in and keeps you there.

Being fully present in your body, grounded, able to let go of what is out there, enables you to go inwards and ask yourself 'What is it that I really want?' instead of leaving it up to your mind (or someone else's mind) to decide for you. Having the capacity to listen to your heart, your intuition, and the patience to wait for the answer instead of thinking and rethinking, can bring you closer to what you actually need, instead of what you think you need.

When it comes to big life choices, being grounded and centred in your body brings you more into the moment. This can really help you get clear on what it is that makes you happy. It can help you stay authentic in knowing what you are good at without feeling like you're bragging. 'I love to make jewellery – I think the pieces I make are really great.' 'I'm good with numbers, but I don't like accounting.'

'Actually, singing is what makes me feel the happiest of all.' You can then make the right choice for all of the aspects of you, and make that choice for yourself instead of trying to do the right thing by everyone else.

> *When you are fully present, you bring*
> *your presence into the world.*

Remember you're here to shine your light, and when you're happy with what you are doing, you shine brighter than at any other time. If you were to hear someone tell you they're really good at something, and they're completely grounded when they say it, you are more likely to believe them than if they're up in their heads. You immediately know if someone is being authentic, because they feel solid and present, substantial, they bring a presence to the room.

Where to next?

I highly recommend that you stay here with the grounding work before jumping into the next chapter. Keep in mind that a tree, if it's not properly grounded, will blow over in the wind. You've become the tree trunk, now you're growing your roots. The next step is to pull down the light. You need to be confident and connected to the Earth before you can expand and grow bigger. Expansion is the subject of the next chapter.

Chapter 5
Expanding

We've talked about Energy Healing, but what we've actually been doing up to this point has been preparation. Yes I know! It's a lot of work to learn how to get centred, and then to learn how to ground yourself. You should really be noticing lots of differences in your energies by the time you get here. Even the act of preparation for healing is healing. In fact, just giving yourself the permission to feel better can work a miracle.

The centring and grounding exercises we have been concentrating on are actually you reorganizing your own biological energy field (biofield). Where you place your attention is where your energies are, so when you centre, you pull the focus of your awareness into your body and become more physically present. When you ground, you bring your Life Force Energy down through your body and into the earth, you connect to the ground so that you are solid, anchored and strong. By reorganizing your biofield you stimulate the natural energy flow in your body, open up the blockages and allow your body to heal itself.

What we are going to do now is 'pull down' Universal Life Force Energy into our biofield for the purposes of healing. This energy is not your own personal Life Force Energy, it comes from the main source of life. It's important to be clear about that. It's like a refreshing bath of light that revives you. It's like stepping into a waterfall of light that fills you up when you feel empty, topping up your natural Divine Source Energy that may be depleted due to the stresses of life.

Like the tree reaching up to the sky, with big strong roots holding it firmly, when we work with this energy, I hope you now understand why we must also be grounded.

Drawing down the energy of healing

Let's take some time now to connect into that higher vibrational source of healing and draw down the energy into your own energy field, so that you can experience it right away.

For this exercise, the intention is for you to connect to the highest vibrational healing energy that you can hold today. This intention is set like this on purpose, because as a vessel for healing energy your body will change every day; some days you can hold more, some days not as much. By asking for the highest vibration that you can hold today, you will always get what you need. You might like to look at an anatomy book at some point to become more familiar with your physical body as it can help you visualize where the light is being sent.

If you feel light-headed from doing this exercise at any time, let go of the imagery around the light, allow your breathing

to come back to its normal breath and let your energies settle. You may need to move your awareness back into your legs, your feet, the ground beneath you, down back down to the tree roots, or even to the crystal cave and check the connection there.

You have to mind yourself, nobody else can, so go gently. If it takes you several sittings with this exercise until you get all the way down to your feet, that's better than not doing it deeply or authentically.

Exercise: healing with high-vibrational energy

❖ Create your space of love. Make sure you're comfortable, warm enough, and that you won't be disturbed.

❖ Breathe. Set your intention to heal, and check in with yourself to see if you're ready to do this work. If you're feeling fear or anxiety, go into it gently and ask what is needed.

❖ Connect with the focus of your awareness. Ask that all of your Life Force Energies come into the space where you are. Wait and feel if there are any energy shifts around this.

❖ Slowly draw the focus of your awareness into your head, then down your body, as before.

❖ Stop at the heart and breathe with it. Imagine the focus of your awareness as a ball of light, and ask it to burn away any heaviness, any grief you may be holding on to.

❖ Now breathe and slowly drop this ball of light down your body with every breath, right down to your pelvis. Split it in two, into your hips and then bring your focus down both legs at the same time.

❖ Move your awareness slowly downwards like a photocopier light scans the glass of the photocopier, scanning down your body, right down your legs into your ankles and feet.

❖ Feel your feet on the ground, connected to the floor.

❖ Go through the floor, down through the building, into the earth, then down through the earth, to the roots of the trees. Visualize these roots. Imagine you are wrapping your energy around a big strong tree root to hold you deep in the earth. Bring your awareness up but leave your energy there.

❖ Bring your awareness back to your heart. Notice how you feel – centred and grounded. Now it's time!

❖ Ask to be connected to the highest vibrational energy of healing that you can hold today. Say it out loud, or feel it in your bones, either way it doesn't matter – this is the intention – to draw down the highest vibrational healing energy that you can hold in your body.

❖ Breathe out any anxiety or fear from your stomach into the ground, through your feet. You're doing great!

❖ Now visualize a bright ball of light about an arm's reach above your head. This is the source of your healing light. It can change colour, sometimes it's gold, sometimes it's pure white, sometimes silver – it knows what you need, so allow it to be whatever it appears to be to you in the moment. Breathe and imagine a cord of light dropping down from this ball of light to the top of your head. Let the energies from this ball of light trickle down the cord, and spill out onto the top of your head. They feel light, bubbly, like champagne.

❖ Imagine champagne bubbles spilling over you, but slowly, much more slowly than real champagne would, spilling over your head,

your forehead, your eyes, your ears, going into your skull, your brain tissue, your blood, into your physical body, the cells, the DNA, healing, purifying, cleansing, clearing you, healing you.

✦ Breathe.

✦ Feel the soft bright light inside you waking up the healthy cells in your body, stimulating growth and flow, opening up all the energy blocks. When the light is in your brain, imagine it softening any tight areas, feeding into the positive thought centres, and visualize light going deep into the parts of your brain that heal and stimulate your physical body, enhancing the nervous connections, healing your communication systems.

✦ Invite this light to come down your body with each breath. Feel this beautiful, bright, healing light coming into your chest, relaxing and opening your chest across your shoulders and down your arms, lighting up your body, lighting up your hands, as if you are made of pure light. Allow this light to drop down into your stomach, softening your stomach, taking away all the anxiety and fear, replenishing the body with healing and rejuvenation. Feel it healing your stomach, your intestines, your liver, your kidneys, your spleen and your pancreas. All your internal organs are blossoming under this beautiful healing light; your body is getting younger.

✦ Breathe the light into your stomach and feel your body fill up with the light. Then, using your intention as you breathe out, 'send' the light down lower into your body, your reproductive organs, your bladder and your colon; send the light into your hips and your pelvis, clearing and cleansing your body, removing all the stress and strain you've been feeling.

✦ Slowly breathe the light into each leg, visualising or imagining your muscles soaking in this healing, nurturing light, becoming healed, tissues repairing, bones glowing with health, the nerves clearing and

all flowing and well. Breathe the light all the way down to your feet. Rest here now.

❖ When you are ready, you can let go of the image of the light, let go of conscious breathing and let your body just breathe and relax. Bring your mind back into the room, become aware of where you are sitting and what is around you. Glow in the light, soften in the light, just be.

❖ When you are ready to come back into the room, feel your feet on the ground, know that you're grounded, press your feet on the floor if it helps. Stretch. Rest. Be.

This can be a very powerful exercise if done consciously, slowly and deeply. The more you practise this, the easier it is to do. This particular exercise can stand you well for years and years without you ever having to change it.

I use this framework for healing every day, several times a day. I don't have to go deeply into every internal organ each time but do a general healing. A quick scan of healing light down my body, just for a pick-me-up! The principle of what I do doesn't change, just the amount of time I spend doing it, and I'm sure that the quality of the 'highest vibrational energy I can hold today' also changes depending on what I eat or drink, how happy I'm feeling, how much work I have to do, it may even depend on the moon cycles.

I do this exercise anywhere I feel I need to. I am able to connect into the ground and then to the healing light pretty quickly, even while waiting in the queue for the bank! See where you can bring it into your day to support

you during your routine. You can do it lying down when you're going to sleep, or when you wake up in the middle of the night and need help getting back to sleep. You can try it whenever you feel anxious. Focus on the exercise instead of the anxiety. Breathe, then let go of the exercise and return to the task you're concentrating on. (If you're highly anxious, you might just want to focus on grounding, as anxiety is a fast moving high-vibrational energy too, and sometimes adding additional high-vibrational energy can make it worse.) Try this exercise before you walk through the door after a hectic day; you can do it in the parked car to calm yourself before going into a family event that may be stressful.

Play with it, have fun with it, keep it light! (Yes light!) The more you do it the more you will notice how you feel, and yes, you might find you are getting more sensitive to energies because you're bringing your awareness to an aspect of your life that you may never have really paid attention to before. It is what it is. I can't say this enough, it's up to you to look after yourself and get help if you need to.

Working with different types of high-vibrational light

There are many different flavours, textures and qualities of light that we can connect to. The beautiful part is that we only know what they are by how they feel to us. Imagine a radio – you can tune in to whichever radio stations you can find by turning the dial, and then when you find your favourites you can programme them in by using a button. We are like the radio, and the high-vibrational frequencies we tune in to are like the radio stations.

As mentioned earlier, some people are born healers, so you could imagine that their radios are top quality and can pick up some stations loud and clear that others never hear at all. That's OK. We all have our own gifts and talents. Imagine this too, that some radio stations are hidden, and to access them we need to be given the frequency to tune in by someone who knows where to find them. For example, Reiki practitioners have to be attuned by a Reiki Master before they can access the energy of Reiki. Attunement is like tuning in to a new radio station.

Let's go back to the analogy using the coffee and filter to represent the quality of healing that an individual can offer. The person as the filter, the life experiences as the coffee granules, the high-vibrational healing energy as the water. But now you are learning that you can have filtered water, tap water and spring water, all different qualities of 'water' as the healing energy. Imagine this – if your coffee granules, your life experiences, are heavy and rough, or have debris in them, no matter what the type of water is, the coffee won't taste good. If your filter is good and strong, and you do your personal work to clear your life experiences, you could be a very powerful healer whether you are attuned to a particular energy or not.

Connecting to a source of unconditional love and light

At the spiritual level we are all made of Life Force Energy, which is the energy of pure, unconditional love. There are no material things at that level so nobody is going to steal from us. There are no physical bodies at that level, so nobody is going to hurt or murder us. At that level, all is made from love.

Like a radio, we can tune in to a higher source of pure, unconditional love, and draw it down into our physical bodies just as we did with the high-vibrational healing light. When you try this exercise, notice how you feel, notice what's different. Notice if you see colours that may be different, if you feel a softness or even if you feel more resistance to the work. And as usual, be slow, be deep, be grounded.

Exercise: connecting to unconditional love for healing

❖ Create your space of love, come into your body and take as much time as you need to fully centre and ground yourself.

❖ Set your intention to experience the energy of unconditional love.

❖ Give permission to do this and notice how your body feels.

❖ Breathe, and if you want to, imagine that you're now tuning in to this energy above your head. Imagine that it is above you now, and then it is entering you through the top of your head, moving down through your body as before.

❖ Breathe, open, experience. Stay for as long as you want, soaking up as much light as you are able.

❖ When you're finished, disconnect from the energy and take as much time as you need to come into balance before moving on with your day.

You can see that the principles are the same, you're just playing with a different energy! What's beautiful about this energy is that it's so supportive and reminds us of our spiritual aspect, that we are made from love, and sometimes we need to remember that.

Try holding in your hand a crystal, such as rose quartz, or a stone, a piece of jewellery or even a candle while you do a healing exercise. When you draw down the healing energy of unconditional love, visualize that it's coming out through your hands and into the object you're holding. You can consciously 'fill' the object up with this beautiful loving energy, and then imagine a white light surrounding the object and sealing all the love into it. You can then wear the jewellery or carry the object with you in your pocket or handbag, or even place it on your desk at work.

This is also a nice thing to do as a gift for someone else, to fill it up with unconditional loving energy, showing that the spiritual aspect of you is honouring the spiritual aspect of your friend, and giving them a present from your heart with no conditions attached!

Working with gratitude as a healing energy

I believe that gratitude has one of the highest vibrations. It's documented that people who make the effort to list five things they are grateful for every day feel happier than those who don't. Recognize that gratitude can be a healing force in your life and try to bring it in more often, feel the burst of lightness that its energy brings.

Exercise: practising gratitude

❖ You don't have to focus on something specific to be grateful for.

Simply say out loud, whisper, or say in your mind:

'Thank you thank you thank you thank you thank you thank you thank you thank you thank you thank you thank you thank you thank

you thank you thank you thank you thank you thank you thank you thank you thank you thank you!'

❖ Can you feel it? If you find this one hard to do, you can focus on a few things you're grateful for. If you're having trouble getting started, begin by saying these statements out loud:

- − 'I am grateful for my body.'
- − 'I am grateful for my breath.'
- − 'I am grateful for this opportunity for life.'
- − 'I am grateful that I have a chance to make a difference to the world.'
- − 'I am grateful for this day.'
- − 'Thank you. Thank you. Thank you!'

You can keep a gratitude journal and list five, or even 10 things you are grateful for every day for a week if you feel called to do so, but make sure each day's list does not contain any repetition from the previous day. You may find it difficult at first, but it gets easier as you access more and more gratitude in yourself.

OK, you're saying, all this gratitude stuff is logical and it's from the headspace, so where's the Energy Healing? Well, thoughts that you are thinking can make you sick, or they can heal. This is you making a conscious choice to create thought forms that are of a high vibration. So it's Energy Healing too. And if you're the type of person who gets caught in negative thought patterns, then breaking the patterns with a gratitude list can be just what you need

in order to change the energy of your mental patterns, leading to healing for the body and soul.

Sending love and light to friends and family

Let's be clear, learning the techniques in this book does not make you a qualified Energy Healing practitioner. I have specifically not included any hand positions for use on other people for that reason. You cannot put a sign up on your door and start charging people for healings unless you undertake professional training, work up client hours and have a mentor to support you. This book does, however, unlock your potential to be a healer and really get you started on a journey of practical healing.

We do have a natural tendency to want to help, so there are ways that you can 'send' healing to other people without placing your hands on them. You need to be clear enough in your Self to make sure that you have a good intention for the healing, no agenda and no attachment to the outcome. If you try this exercise and the person to whom you have chosen to send the energy feels much better, please know that it was a combination of your intention and their permission to receive the healing – the magic happens somewhere outside us, the miracle is when everything opens and expands. You don't 'do' anything – so you can't take credit for any healing that may happen. But you can create ripples, and from the ripples can come great transformation.

For this exercise you can send love and light to someone who you know, whether they are a relative or friend, live near you or far away. Asking their permission directly is

best, so they know that it's coming. However, you can send the healing to them without asking their brain, but using the yes/no technique to ask their energy: 'Do I have permission to send (name of person) healing today?' If you get a 'no', then the answer is no, and you must respect that. By respecting it, it means you are more likely to get a 'yes' the next time. Don't be forceful in your mind's eye. Be gentle, as if you're offering dessert after a lovely dinner, and don't be insulted if someone says they don't want any.

The first part of this exercise can take 10 minutes or more depending on what kind of 'zone' you're in. Please remember that you need to send the love and light from an unemotional space, a place of no agenda and pure love. This is difficult if you're emotional yourself, if you are caught up in stress or a conflict, or you are grieving. You don't want this amazing gift of healing travelling to your loved one wrapped up in your heavy emotions, just as you wouldn't want to receive the same from them. If it doesn't feel right to send it, then respect your intuition and don't send it until you are feeling better.

Exercise: sending love and light

❖ Go to your space of love, take the time to ground yourself, centre and connect to your healing light.

❖ Breathe.

❖ Draw down the healing light so that you've got a flow in your body, feel the energy flowing around you and allow your personal energy space to expand.

❖ Set your intention – who is this love and light for? Picture them in your mind, and see a soft glow around them. Ask them in your mind's eye if they would like to receive healing light from you. Wait to feel a 'yes' or a 'no' from your intuition, your felt sense, not your brain.

❖ If you do get a 'no', perhaps leave it for another time, or choose someone else. You can still send a burst of love to them, like the Energy Healing ball, just to say something like 'I love you and I understand and it's here for you if you want it'.

❖ Focus on the person you have a 'yes' for.

❖ Imagine they are surrounded by a bubble of energy, and see the edges of this bubble become more permeable, getting ready to receive the love and light that you want to send to them.

❖ Be aware of your body and what is going on with the energy around you. Slow down your thoughts and become aware of your breath. Focus on your breath, hear your heart beating and feel the ground beneath your feet, and begin to breathe from your stomach.

❖ Place your hands on your stomach and feel it rise and fall as you breathe. Relax your stomach and let any tension flow out and down your legs, and into the earth. Become centred in your body, feel your legs and your lower body open, and send all the tension you carry downwards and to the floor. Stay doing this for a while until you really feel that you are in a place of stillness.

❖ Bring your awareness to your heart. Visualize it. Is it closed or open? Is it small or large? What colour is it? Breathe into your heart and imagine the colours getting stronger, your heart expanding in size and opening. It is radiating love, like sunbeams.

❖ Imagine that the sunbeams radiating out of your heart are stretching into your body and filling it with love and light. Stay there breathing

for a while and let the love and light clear away any negativity or unwanted emotional energy from your own energy space.

❖ Imagine now that you are a clear channel of love and light. As you imagine your sunbeams getting bigger, and visualize your own energy expanding and filling the room with love and light. If you get light-headed doing this, check you are still grounded, and perhaps dissolve away a little bit of the intensity of your light, until you come more into balance with it.

❖ Connect in with the image of the person you've chosen to work with. Imagine the sunbeams are beaming out from you, going into the space between you and them, and reaching them wherever they are, reaching their energy field, connecting into their energy and washing them too – with pure, unconditional love and light.

❖ As you breathe, you can expand and imagine your love and light even stronger, filling them up, relaxing them, healing them. Imagine their face softening, their shoulders dropping, their breath slowing down, their body relaxing and them feeling more present and grounded.

❖ When you feel ready to stop, you can reduce the intensity of the light you're sending out and imagine that the person you've sent it to gently disconnects from you, that the bubble they're in gets less permeable and they are sealed up and protected and safe.

❖ Travel with your sunbeams of light through space and time and back into the room that you are in, back to your physical body. If you are feeling you've still got more to give, choose one other person who may need love and light today. They may be someone you know or they may be a stranger. I like to use this part of the exercise to work with someone I'm having difficulty with, someone I know is unhappy and wanting to pick a fight with me, or someone I'm not getting along with.

✦ Start with the question – do you want healing? Wait for the 'yes' or the 'no' – trust that even someone you may be fighting with will accept healing from you if it's given with no agenda. (You're not healing them so that they like you better or so that you win the argument!!) Once you get the go-ahead, spread out your healing sunbeams, connect in with their energy, wherever they may be across space and time, and visualize them relaxing and opening up to healing. Visualize them relax and smile as they feel warm and loved, and maybe imagine the anger between you dissolving away.

✦ When you are ready, let all the images dissolve slowly and come back into your space of love. Bring yourself back into your body, breathing slowly.

✦ This is a powerful exercise, and when you send healing to someone it amplifies the healing that you receive, so make sure you take as much time as you need before running off and doing something else after this!

✦ Feel your arms, your legs, your feet in your shoes, feel that you are here, in your physical body, connected to the ground. Wiggle your fingers. Feel like you have completely disconnected from the people you were working with, in a gentle, loving way.

✦ When you are ready, open your eyes.

It could be fun to call or text the person you worked with after you've finished and see how they feel or what they experienced. It's wonderful to experience receiving healing from someone else this way too. The results are sometimes surprising and unexpected.

The healing ball of light

Sometimes it's fun to mix things up a little bit, to try things in a different way. This healing ball exercise is light and playful and for this reason you don't have to spend heaps of time grounding and centring first. It can do two things – it can fill you with light, or it can lift off the energies that don't belong to you, or that are weighing you down.

Exercise: creating a healing ball of light

✦ Ask to be connected to a high-vibrational healing light. Imagine this light comes through the top of your head, down to your chest and heart, and then spills up and over your shoulders and down your hands.

✦ Cup your hands and place them facing each other, and imagine the healing light pooling in the space in the middle, creating a ball of light.

✦ Wait for a bit as it builds up, then you can take the ball of light and put it straight into your body. If you're in pain, say, you could put it directly into the spot where it hurts. Or you could imagine that you're rolling the ball of light up and down your body, and the ball of light is pulling up and out of your body the heavy and old energies that you don't need, while the flow from the healing light at the top of your head is replacing them with the good, high-vibrational ones.

✦ You might want to imagine you're rolling it about particularly on your chest around your heart centre if you're feeling upset or angry with someone, and give yourself permission to let go of the energies that are weighing you down.

❖ You could also imagine someone to whom you want to send healing, and imagine you 'throw' the ball of light through space and time to them. The ball could be bigger than them by the time it reaches them so that they are completely absorbed by the light, or you could imagine that they catch the ball and place it where they feel they need it most.

So you can see there are many applications for this healing ball. You can even imagine that you throw the ball up into space, and then send it back in time to yourself when you were upset or experiencing a difficult situation. You can imagine that you're sending it ahead of yourself into the future, so you know that you're supporting yourself. For example, if you're going somewhere stressful, such as an interview, or it's a day when something unavoidable is happening, such as a court date or even a wedding! You can imagine this healing ball to be very big in the present time – bigger than you – and then imagine yourself stepping into it so you feel more protected or supported for a couple of hours. See how many different ways you can apply this exercise to your own life. And have fun with it!

How do you feel?

This is a question I ask clients a lot, because it's so important.

Let's take a breather here so you can check in with yourself. You're at a point now where you have the skills you need to do a great job healing yourself.

Look back on all the work you have done since picking up this book. Notice how you feel now – what's different? Was

it what you expected? Was it better or worse? Think about what you have learned, about what questions this work has stirred up for you.

Your life is a journey, so question everything. You don't have to settle for OK, when fantastic is available to you. You just might have to work a little bit harder to get there.

Here are a few questions to think about at this point:

1. What drew you to Energy Healing in the first place?

2. Now that you've experienced it, what is it that you think it will heal for you?

3. Are you willing to put in the time to develop a daily practice of healing?

4. Can you do all this on your own or do you need to ask for help?

Remember the swimming pool image, with the dye? Well, now you've started to pour in the fresh water with this exercise, clearing out the old, bringing in the new, but it takes time. I don't want you to have an expectation of when you will be 'healed' because that may never happen. There will always be more things to throw you off course, to challenge you, to make you grow, because that's what life is about. Healing is a process of clearing over time, instead of something that's a quick fix. Yes, you can have spontaneous deep transformational healing, but often before that happens you need a slower process of preparation for that healing. Healing is never finished as long as you have a physical body.

The next section of the book is about how you can apply Energy Healing to your life. I talk about things you can do to bring it into your day, ways to heal your environment, and the impact your healing has on your family. I will look at how to create a daily spiritual practice using Energy Healing, so that you always feel connected and balanced in your life.

You may want to stop here and work with what you've got so far, to deepen it, and that's perfect. You might want to read on and do it all, or come back in a few weeks or a few months to embrace the third part of the book. It's all good.

Listen to your heart, to your intuition – it will guide you on your right path.

Part III

TAKING IT FURTHER

'There are only two ways to live your life. One is as though nothing is a miracle. The other is as though everything is a miracle.'
ALBERT EINSTEIN

Chapter 6

Creating more space
for your Self

Now that you're working on your biological energy field, you will be getting bigger! Not bigger as in putting on weight, but your actual energy field will be expanding. Your vibration will change, your outlook on life may also change, and you will feel more relaxed and confident in your decision-making as you're better able to connect to your heart and your intuition.

You might also find that certain things that you used to 'put up with' become much more difficult to tolerate. As you expand, small things like the electrical hum from the fridge or static from the television may begin to irritate you more than before. Because you are now more aware of your energy sensitivities you may notice this, but it's also possible that you were that sensitive the whole time. By bringing your focus of awareness into your body *and* your energy, you're discovering more and more about how you are made.

In order to support yourself fully as you expand, you also need to allow your idea of who you are to expand. Let me explain this through a client's story.

Sonia worked in a university as one of the Administrators for a busy Science department. When she came to see me her energy field was contracted, she was catching colds all the time and she was both physically and mentally exhausted. Our first session was pure Energy Healing as she wasn't able to talk about how she was feeling.

After the session she said, 'It's like I was all hunched over and small, like an old lady, and now I feel much taller again. I didn't even realize how small I felt.'

She went home and slept for eight hours. When she came for session two she was sleeping better, feeling brighter and not as tired. But she was finding herself getting agitated frequently.

'By the time it's 3 p.m. I've had enough, and I have another three hours of the day left to go! The phone really annoys me, and when there are students in a queue, lecturers wanting my attention and the phone rings, I want to scream! It never bothered me so much before, I guess I was just tuning everything out.'

Here's the thing – you can't function if you get extremely agitated or upset by these things. Remember, just because you notice them now and are more aware of their impact on you doesn't mean that you are going to be upset by them forever. By bringing the focus of your awareness into

your energy and consciously expanding yourself outwards, it's as if you have more space to hold all of these things, and you can breathe and manage it all much better.

Exercise: focusing your awareness

❖ Bring the focus of your awareness into your body and feel your feet on the ground. Notice how you feel. Now breathe.

❖ You are going to use your intention to tell your energy field to open and expand.

❖ First, check in with yourself to see where you are with it. Use the image of the bud of a flower opening up, or a butterfly opening out its wings and shaking them off before flying, or a crumpled piece of paper that opens up and smooths out. Is there an image that suits you better? What is it?

❖ With this image in mind, let it show you how expanded or contracted you actually are in this moment.

❖ When you feel in alignment with the image, then breathe into it and relax. You are the flower opening, you are the butterfly stretching out its wings, the piece of paper unfolding.

❖ Breathe. Relax and imagine you're releasing all the blocks to opening up.

❖ Stay with it until you feel an improvement.

❖ The situation hasn't changed, but you have. What feels different now?

After teaching this technique to Sonia she told me how she was able to apply it at work.

'At about 3 p.m. last Thursday I did the yes/no technique, and asked myself if my energies had contracted. The answer was a big 'yes!' I love sunflowers, so I used the image of a sunflower opening to help me open up my energy again. I know we used a rose in session, but a sunflower felt more like me in that moment. It took a while, as I didn't force the flower to open. Instead I used my breathing and connected into my feet and the ground while smiling and nodding to the students! After a few breaths I felt something loosen inside me and then I was able to open up, I felt a burst of light shine through me and I felt bigger and taller – just like I did during our session. It was remarkable! I could do it myself!! When I brought my attention more fully back to work, it was busy but I was able to handle it. I didn't lose my temper and the phone didn't seem to grate on me so much. By 5:30 p.m. I was still bright and happy, and even my colleagues noticed a difference in me!'

The only thing that changed in Sonia's day was Sonia. When she was big in her energies she had more space for herself, and the demands that work made on her didn't impact her in the same way. She was a tall sunflower reaching towards the sun, pulling down the light, standing up strong and holding her own, instead of a small, depleted and hunched-over version of herself.

The main problem people have with the Energy Healing techniques is remembering to do them! If a sunflower is your thing, you could wear a yellow bracelet, put a picture of a sunflower on your phone or as your desktop wallpaper,

or place a miniature sunflower at your desk or even a small framed image of one, so you have a visual reminder to do the exercise when you need to. Change the images frequently so you don't get too used to them and forget what they signify. You can get creative with it!

Getting 'big' can protect you from danger

Just as we can 'get big' to create more space for ourselves so we can manage life better, we also can 'get big' to connect into our source of power and strength to feel protected and strong.

Although he's less than five feet tall, David has a strong presence and understands the basic principles of Energy Healing.

'When I go home from work at night, I have to walk down a dark alleyway and it sometimes makes me nervous. What I've started doing lately is making my energy 'big' as I walk home. In fact, I imagine that my energy is like a tank – impenetrable. I've noticed that I'm not so nervous any more as I walk, and nobody has approached me.'

We know when someone is angry or happy just by how their energy feels, we also know if someone is vulnerable or weak. By deliberately and intentionally being big and strong in his energy, David is telling the world 'Don't mess with me,' and the world responds to that by not messing with him!

I was working with Martha, a 14-year-old girl who was being bullied at school. She had shrunk down into

a smaller version of herself due to repeated verbal attacks from three boys in her class. It took a while in session for her to expand and relax her energy as she was upset and very contracted. Once she was able to expand, we worked on grounding so that she could feel connected to the earth. We often need something for our brains to work on that complements the work we do with our energy. We used an affirmation that captured the energy she needed in those moments when she felt threatened. 'You do not have any power over me, I am safe.'

Affirmations are very powerful when used in an energetic way, rather than just saying them because they sound good! You've got to mean them. You've got to believe them, and then feel them inside your core.

Martha and I worked on this affirmation to make sure that she really knew the bullies had no actual power over her, they couldn't really hurt her and that she was, in fact, safe.

*'I saw the boys coming over to me at break time, like they always do, only this time I had my secret weapon affirmation! I said it to myself a few times and then I was able to look them in the eye. I grew bigger like we did in session, and pretended I was that big marble statue on **Game of Thrones** – as big as a city – so that my energy was even bigger than the three boys put together! They didn't attack me that time. They seemed a bit confused! It was great fun and I felt brilliant afterwards!'*

Nothing changed in that situation except for Martha. She switched from being a victim to being empowered. The bullies didn't like this, and unfortunately, after they regrouped, they decided to fight back even harder. This is a normal thing, the last hurrah – the test to see if the change is real, and the anger because they don't want to lose. This is similar to a healing crisis. Sometimes things do get worse before they get better. When the bullies hit back harder than ever, Martha was energized because she knew what worked the last time and she held her ground – knowing they had no power over her, staying big in her energy. She also discovered that as bad as their taunting was before, when she felt big and strong she didn't get upset the way she used to. She laughed at them! Martha was no longer a victim. The bullies were no longer getting what they wanted from her so they had to move on.

Getting big doesn't mean putting on weight!

When we talk about getting big our brain immediately thinks that means putting on physical weight. Subconsciously, some people overeat because they want to be physically big as a form of protection. If you start using these exercises and begin to expand and strengthen your energy when you feel unsafe, you might find that your need for food – if you relate to this – decreases as you become more confident working with your energy. The more work you do on yourself using these techniques, the more comfortable you'll become with the size of your energy, and the less likely it will be that you'll need to fill yourself up with food, instead of healing energy.

Exercise: working with your energy to avoid comfort-eating

❖ Next time you find yourself eating for comfort, take a moment to breathe before you eat to break the pattern. Ask yourself: 'Is this food for my body?'

❖ Get an answer, then breathe and ask, 'Does my brain need this food?' Wait for an answer, and then ask, 'Can I heal this with Energy Healing?'

❖ If the answer is 'yes', put down the food, place one hand on your heart and the other on your stomach, then draw down healing energy for a few minutes until you feel more balanced.

❖ You may also want to ask yourself: 'Do I need to get help for this?'

Healing and your family system

We're talking about space and expanding, and when you change your shape, you affect everyone that's connected to you.

Imagine your family system is a bit like the solar system. Each member of your family is a planet that spins at its own speed, on its own axis. Some planets are bigger than others, some planets spin faster than others – get the picture? You're at the centre, and each of these planets not only spins in its own way, but it then also spins around you. Some of them are closer to you than others, and some of these planets come in fast and leave as quickly as they came.

It might be fun to draw out your family system with you at the centre, using lots of different colours so that you

can visualize it more clearly. I use this as an exercise in workshops and people are amazed at how their pictures turn out; they see patterns in their family system that they never realized were there before. If you imagine you were small in your energy for years, the system shaping itself around you, but then, after connecting into healing energy you get bigger, you can imagine that some adjustments may have to be made.

Sarah had been diagnosed with bipolar disorder early in her life. Her parents were both alcoholics and became violent when they were drunk, and so Sarah and her sister, Patricia, moved in together to start a life of their own when they were in their early 20s. But a pattern had developed between the two sisters, in which Sarah would have mood swings, panic attacks and bouts of depression and Patricia would comfort her, cook her meals and make sure she took her medication. She came to see me after several years of living like this, wanting to improve her life. I taught her some Energy Healing techniques and she started doing them every day. On the third session with me it was apparent that something had changed.

'Patricia is angry at me. I don't know what I did. She won't stop picking on me, she's nasty, angry and screams all the time – I stand there and shake in front of her. It's like my world is falling apart – I don't know what to do.'

'How are you feeling in yourself?' I asked her.

'After our last session I went home and slept for 12 hours. When I woke up I felt brighter, more positive,

*had more energy. I tried the meditation you gave me
every day for the next week, and I was able to do it.
I felt much calmer for a while, but now this fighting
with Patricia is really horrible and I think it's making
me sick again – do you think she's angry because I'm
getting better?'*

A codependent relationship develops when someone is
sick and the other is the caregiver. As Sarah got better
she needed less and less care from Patricia, and Patricia
felt rejected and abandoned, and lashed out at Sarah.
Sarah was not strong enough to manage the situation, and
unfortunately she stopped coming for healing so as not to
upset her sister further.

It's important for you to know as you go deeper into your
healing process that your healing will affect your entire
family. Sometimes it's in a good way; where there is no
codependency in a family, they're delighted and pleased
to see someone feeling better and becoming happy. But
sometimes there's jealousy, there's anger and resentment.
Patricia was not ready to heal yet, and she didn't want
Sarah to heal because it was going to force her to do work
she didn't want to do. There may be people in your family
too, who by seeing your progress may become unhappy,
knowing that they have work to do as well.

The next few exercises are designed to help you manage
the shifts in your family system as you grow and heal.
However, your healing may bring up deeper issues either
in you or in your family that cannot be managed simply
by using the exercises in this book. Do consider getting
additional help and support if you need to.

You also need to know that you are connected energetically to everyone you care about, and anyone who cares about you, even if they are not blood relations. They may not be in your actual family, but they are in an energy system with you, similar to the family system I've described, and they can also feel the impact as your energy shifts and heals.

> *I had a client come for one session of pure Energy Healing. About 15 minutes into the session his phone rang, and rang. The fifth time it rang I brought it over to him and asked him to turn it off. When the session was over he looked at the phone and there were nine missed calls and five text messages, all from his ex-girlfriend.*
>
> *'She must be angry at you for clearing your energy so you can move on with your life!' I said.*
>
> *'Oh my gosh!' he said. 'Now I understand why she's been acting weird all week! Yes, I met someone else. I'm ready to move on.'*

Creating more space for yourself in your family system

In this exercise, we work within the family system to reorganize it, so you have more space for yourself. Read through it carefully before you try it so that you know what to expect. After doing this exercise a few times don't be surprised if your brother phones you, or your cousin!

Exercise: healing your family system

❖ Sit in your space of love, breathe and come into your body.

❖ Wait until you feel you are fully present in the room.

❖ Bring the focus of your awareness into your head, and with every breath, drop down deeper into your body.

❖ Bring yourself all the way in, and down to your stomach. Notice how you are feeling, if you are fearful or anxious, and know that you're not hurting anyone doing this, you're just reorganizing the energy around you so there's more room for your new healed self.

❖ Bring your awareness into your hips, and move it down your legs slowly, feeling like they're opening up as you move down each leg into your knees, into your ankles, then into your feet.

❖ Bring your awareness down through the floor and ground yourself as deep as you need to go. When you feel secure and grounded, bring your awareness back up to your body, to your heart centre.

❖ Now draw down healing energy from above your head; take as long as you need to clear anything that needs to leave before you can continue this exercise. Expand your energy field outwards so that you are big, bright and shining in your mind's eye, and you fill the space you are in. How do you feel now?

❖ Imagine you are the centre of your family system. Don't imagine them all at once, start with the person that you feel closest to in your family. See them as a ball of light separate to you, but yet inside your energy field. They could be to the left of you, to the right, above you, below you, in front of you or behind you. What colour are they? How close are they to you? Are they bigger than you? Smaller than you? How fast do they spin? What does it feel like to imagine them there?

❖ Be with it however it feels for a while, just to gauge that it feels the way things actually are and not how you may think things are. Once you're ready, take a breath and imagine that on your next out breath you're gently pushing this ball of light, this family member, gently outside your energy field. Now do it. Slowly. Know that they're not gone, they're just that bit further away from you to give you space. How does this feel? Have you moved them far enough away? If not, on the next breath push them out a little bit more. Is that better? Keep going until you feel like you have enough space for yourself.

❖ Dissolve the images away, and take a moment to come into balance. Now imagine someone else from your family – where do they appear in your energy field? Does the position of the first person change just by imagining this person? Observe, and when you feel grounded and centred in yourself, use your breath again to gently push the ball of light outwards, away from you, until it feels right.

❖ Now you feel much bigger in your space, in your energy, stretch your body if you need to.

❖ Who else do you need to shift out of your energy field? Let them come into your mind's eye, and repeat it again. It might be someone you don't expect, so check with the yes/no technique and trust your instinct. Perhaps three is enough for one sitting, perhaps you feel like you want to keep going. Stay grounded and slow while you work.

❖ To finish, you can create a healing ball of light between your hands, fill it up with unconditional love and light, and then allow it to grow so big that it's the same size as you. Then grow it bigger still, so that it touches the people in your family system who you've shifted out of your space. Send love and light to each of them, and if you feel like you need to talk to them, do it here, to their energy, in this safe space. Say thank you, and tell them you love them. Tell them how

you feel when they do what they do, and ask them please not to do it any more. Know that you are healing the family when you do this, and know that some people in your family are not ready for healing. It's all as it should be.

❖ Now let all the images dissolve away. Bring your awareness back to your physical body and your breath. Feel your feet on the ground, and feel the chair beneath you.

❖ Take time to come back into your space of love, and be gentle on yourself. This is big work. Well done.

———

This *is* big work, I'm not kidding. You might feel tired after this one, and you might find that after a day or two the system slips back to the way it was, and that you have to do it again. One of my clients did this exercise with me and two days later his mother phoned and screamed at him for an hour and then hung up on him. She didn't remember a word she had said when he asked her about it the next time they met up, but thankfully, he was prepared, so he didn't take it personally!

Remember you can use the exercises from Chapter 5 in combination with this one – sending a healing ball of light to someone, or sending love and light directly to the person you have in mind. Shrink the family system in your mind's eye and send the whole system a healing ball of light. Play with it! It is serious, but be light in it. If you find working with your family invokes anger in you, take your anger outside these exercises and deal with it there so it doesn't destroy all the good work you are doing.

Check in on your family system in your mind's eye from time to time to see if it's shifted back. Make little tweaks to your own energy space now and then to ensure that you don't feel encroached upon by Aunty Violet, or by Granny May! Only work with how they interact with you, don't worry about how they are interacting with each other. That's their business and not yours. If you respect their boundaries, they are more likely to respect yours in return.

❖ ❖ ❖

Energy Healing for the office

If you work in an office you may be in a space that you don't really have much control over. Whether you work for yourself or for someone else, chances are you are restricted in some ways as to how much you can do with your workspace. You may be sitting beside someone who irritates you, or you may even be doing work that you don't enjoy. You may be at the beck and call of a manager's mood swings, or working on a project with a group of people with whom you feel you cannot be yourself. Just like some of the other examples in this chapter, the situation might not be likely to change, but you can. You can bring Energy Healing into these situations to help you expand and ground yourself, clear your head and bring strength and focus into your day.

Exercise: creating a healed space for your desk

You can create an oasis of healing energy at your desk if you put your mind to it! I used to have many people come up just to say 'Hello' when I worked in a busy office, because they always felt better in the energy space I created!

Here are some practical ideas to clear the heavy energies of your space and raise the vibration:

❖ Put something on your desk that makes you smile. You could try making the healing crystal from Chapter 5.

❖ Always have fresh flowers or a plant nearby.

❖ See if you can move extension cables with plugs away from where you are sitting.

❖ Try and have as much natural light as possible. Change a normal light bulb for a full-spectrum light bulb if you can.

❖ Put up a picture or some artwork that makes your heart happy. If you can't hang it on the wall, you could use it for your desktop wallpaper.

❖ Keep your space organized. Is there a lot of clutter on your desk? Can you file the paperwork away and have a tidy desk?

You get the idea. While these are not directly Energy Healing ideas, everything affects the energy around you and you can change big energies by changing small things.

Remember to get big at work

You don't feel the physical impact of people's emotional energy as much when you are expanded in your energies. Offices are great places for gossip, for heavy emotional energies of fear, anxiety, jealousy, competitiveness and resentment (remember Sandra in Chapter 2?).

Check in with yourself during the day and remember to get big; imagine other people's emotional energies slide off you and into the ground. Breathe them out if they feel stuck, and get big and strong like we've done already. Use your desktop wallpaper to remind you that you can get big like a tree, like a sunflower or like a statue.

Consciously expanding and feeling big at work can also help you feel more grounded at meetings, interviews or presentations. It can help you access your intuition and make better decisions. Ask yourself the yes/no questions about work issues! You've done the work already – just remember to apply it to the situations where it can be most helpful to you.

Exercise: healing at the end of the working day

You might have picked up other people's energy during your day at work and you don't want to bring it home, especially if it's stress around work or money. This type of emotional energy can 'stick' to you and because it's similar to what you may have experienced before, you think it's yours. You need to clear it away from your energy so that you don't get caught up in it, or pass it on to someone else. Take a few minutes at the end of your working day to try this:

❖ Breathe, centre and ground.

❖ Connect to a source of healing light.

❖ Breathe it down and into your body, relax and expand.

❖ Imagine that as you expand, any emotional energies that do not belong to you are melting away, dissolving away, falling into the ground.

❖ Ask for all energies that are not yours to leave, just to emphasize your intention.

❖ You can also ask for any healing that you may need before going home.

❖ Give thanks for the day that you had, for the evening to come and for a good night's sleep.

You can do this at your desk after you switch off your computer, or in the car before you start the engine. Taking a few minutes every day to clear the energies from work is so beneficial. It enables you to return home feeling more refreshed and grateful for all the good in your life.

❖ ❖ ❖

Raising the vibration in your home

Just as you can make an oasis at work, you can bring fresh eyes into your living space and find ways to raise the energy there, too. Clutter is a big issue. If you can remove clutter, you open space for new energies to come in. I'm not an expert at Feng Shui, but if you felt drawn to it, you might consider getting a Feng Shui practitioner to come in and help reorganize the flow in your home so that you can invite

in more wealth, happiness or romance. This may involve moving mirrors on to different walls, or putting plants in certain corners of the house. It's a whole science in itself, and whether you seek an expert or not, clearing clutter and keeping your living space tidy and organized will certainly help keep your vibration high. See the Resources on (*page 163*) for more information.

Consider doing the following:

❖ Remove clutter. Clean away stale dirt and dust.

❖ Paint in fresh, bright colours, upgrade your curtains, get a bright throw for the sofa/bed, buy in some new cushions or a new duvet.

❖ Remove anything from plain sight that makes you emotional (such as a photo of a loved one who has died).

❖ Use aromatherapy candles/incense/oils to bring in smells that you love.

❖ Remove the television and any electrical equipment from your bedroom or sleeping area.

❖ Replace bulbs with natural light spectrum bulbs, use timers to switch off electrical appliances, replace old appliances such as microwaves, kettles and toasters for newer, more economical models.

You don't have to do any of these things, simply do what you feel moved to do, as you feel moved to do it. It's all common sense; remove anything that makes you feel heavy and slow, and bring in new things that make you feel lighter in your Self. You can use the 'yes/no' exercise if you're not sure of something.

Exercise: raising the vibration of a room

You can apply this healing exercise to any room you like. You can even do it in the office if you feel safe to do so. I love doing this in a hotel room because it makes me feel like the room is clearer for me, instead of containing the energies of all the people that may have slept in it before I got there!

❖ Standing up, face a corner of the room and connect into the ground.

❖ Ask to be connected to the highest vibration of healing light that you can hold today.

❖ Visualize the light entering your body, coming down your arms and out of your hands.

❖ Fill the walls with this healing energy from a distance by moving your hands slowly, up and down the wall, as if you are painting them with healing energy. Imagine that the healing energy from you is clearing away anything of low vibration.

❖ When you've finished the first wall, turn and do the next, and the next and so on. If there is a window, do that too.

❖ When you've finished the walls, then use your intention to send healing into the ceiling, and then to the floor.

❖ You might like to finish by placing your hands on yourself, sitting down and just breathing as the light continues to flow through your body.

❖ Stay grounded!

Energy Healing on a 'needs' basis

How else do you think you can apply the principles of Energy Healing to your life? Are there other areas that I've not mentioned here in which it would be suitable for you to feel more empowered by getting big in your energies? For example you could apply the 'family systems' exercise to projects at work that are getting on top of you. Visualize the project you're working on and then push it out of your energy field when you go home so it doesn't preoccupy you all evening! Don't be any less gentle with this than you would be with a family member; you don't know who is connected to this project and the energy of the project itself might get damaged if you do it too roughly!

Many of these exercises are ready to use in your daily life, but they're on a 'needs' basis rather than something you need to do every day. In the next chapter we will look more deeply at how you can bring Energy Healing into your life as a daily spiritual practice, taking you further down the road of healing.

Chapter 7

Energy Healing as a spiritual practice

It's more than likely you already have a spiritual practice, you just may not realize it.

What is a spiritual practice?

Anything that helps you connect to your Spirit, helps you feel better, calmer, more relaxed and happy, can be considered a spiritual practice. It's a practice because it's never done, never finished, you keep doing it. The intention for a practice is to be mindful rather than on autopilot – to have your focus of awareness fully present so you can experience your practice fully, deeply and wholeheartedly.

Setting a specific routine for a spiritual practice might be too ambitious if it doesn't suit your lifestyle. You don't have to spend 20 minutes in meditation every morning if it's too big a commitment. If you can do it, great, but if it's more than likely that you won't be able to do it, you may spend the day feeling bad about not doing it, which defeats the purpose in the first place. A spiritual practice should be

manageable and something that you enjoy and can do anytime you want, whenever you feel you need it.

Why do we need a spiritual practice?

When I ask my clients if they have a daily spiritual practice some of them look at me sideways, as if I'm speaking a foreign language. For me, a daily spiritual practice is vital for good health. Taking time out every day to reconnect with yourself is like a reset, it helps you get your priorities back in the right order instead of allowing yourself to drift and the energies around you to magnify your fears and doubts.

We do so many things on autopilot that we may not even be aware that we are doing them. For example, I always used to forget if I'd locked my car when I'd parked it. Then when I was miles away, my heart would leap up into my chest, and I'd be worried, 'Did I lock the car?' I'd never remember! I've lost count of the number of times I had to go back to the car just to check it! I now mindfully lock my car every time I park by stopping for a moment before I walk away and bringing my attention and awareness to it. Sometimes I even say 'I am locking the car now' as I lock it. From time to time I'll still ask myself if I have locked the car, and I can say for certain the answer is always 'yes'. Once we have awareness, we are present, and we have a choice. The key is to get the awareness.

The problem is, when we tune out our mind tends to wander, we lose awareness of what we are doing and we tend to gravitate towards the things that are upsetting us. By doing this, we are feeding our energy and awareness

into things we don't actually want to grow. Pulling our energy back from wandering thoughts, from what we are feeding, is so important, and if we incorporate this into a daily practice, we get better at doing it.

We live in a community, not in isolation

We are surrounded by people, and whether we spend time with them every day or not, we still get affected by them. For the most part, people are not responsible for their emotional energies and tend to 'dump' them on other people and walk away. I'm sure you've experienced this. It's not that people do it on purpose, they just don't know what else to do. If we can check in with ourselves every day, clear what is not ours and reorganize what is, it stops a build-up over time, which can make us sick.

> *'I met with the girls for lunch. It was the usual chatter, but Rosemary was very quiet. I knew something was wrong, so I asked her, and she burst into tears. She told us that she thought her boyfriend was going to break up with her. We held her hand and listened as she went over all the things that were going on in her head. When she was finished, her eyes were brighter, and she looked better, but I felt tired. When I went out of the restaurant, I felt a heaviness in my chest, and it stayed there all day, in fact, now that I think of it, it didn't lift from me until after dinner.'*

Does this sound familiar? It's not that Rosemary knowingly dumped her emotional pain onto her friend, but her friend wanted to look after her so naturally she took it on, and she went home with it. Rosemary felt better, but her friend didn't.

When we are on autopilot, if our thoughts are feeding the fears and the doubts, we resonate with the fears and the doubts, and are more likely to pick up on other people's fears and doubts too. Studies in positive psychology have shown that we have a tendency to feel more stressed when we are surrounded by stressful things such as media reports or violence on television. So even if we are not surrounded by people, we can be surrounded by media that affects us in the same way.

We also prefer to go with the crowd rather than stand out from it. Our basic nature wants to help, too, so we have a tendency to get drawn into feelings, behaviours and stories that belong to the group, rather than to us as individuals. In Ireland, where I live, people love a good story, and they tell it and tell it and tell it again, so much so that the story itself takes on a life and an energy of its own. When the story is about murder or suicide, war or epidemics, the stories can take more and more of our energies away from us and we contract our biofield, and feel smaller and smaller and less able to function.

Having a spiritual practice reminds us of who we are

It's time to recognize that if we take on other energies that are not ours we can drown under the weight of them. We also need to recognize that if we give everything of ourselves away to everyone else, we have nothing left to give. A daily practice is vital to remind us of what belongs to us and what does not, and it gives us an opportunity to reconnect to our intuition and raise our vibration. This is being responsible for our energies, and as I said above,

most people are not responsible, so perhaps now it's time to take responsibility and just do it. Every day. It's not that you are going to change the world by having a spiritual practice, but it's more likely you will be able to find happiness and balance in your own life if you do.

We have a tendency to take on other people's heavy energies.

We also have a tendency to give our energies away to other people, situations, fears and emotional/physical pain.

We need to take our energies back, clear them and heal them, so we can come into balance and stay healthy.

Just as a car needs petrol so it can keep driving, our Life Force Energy is the fuel that drives us. We need to take time every day to take back our energies from areas that are draining them, to feed and clear them of other people's needs and wants, and to heal them to raise their vibration. When we do this, we come into alignment, resonate with peace, joy and love and are at our best.

How to create your own daily spiritual practice

In order to create your own spiritual practice, you need to choose something you enjoy, something that can fit into your day, and something that doesn't feel like a mountain to climb! I've outlined some ideas here that you might like to try. Give them a go and see what works best for you.

If you want more inspiration, do come and visit me on Facebook, Twitter, Pinterest or my blog, as I regularly share exercises and meditations that people find very helpful. I

also hold online classes in which I help you create your own daily spiritual practice. You can tell me how you get on with these exercises and share your experiences with others on social media.

Bringing all the pieces together

Before we start creating our own daily spiritual practice, let's take a quick review of what we have learned so far, so you know what you have to work with.

Your energy is not always in your body: You found the focus of your awareness, brought it into your body, and felt how different that is to the normal way we live, with our Life Force Energy being mostly outside our bodies, up around our minds. Let's change that, and have 'being centred' as the new normal!

You function best when you are centred: You then learned how to centre yourself properly by bringing the focus of your awareness down through your body, connecting into your heart. This is invaluable as it really helps you feel more contained in your body. It feeds your body with more energies too, so you are healthier, and have a good connection to your intuition and a clear way of getting a yes or no answer.

When you are grounded you stay in your body: You brought your energy connection down to Mother Earth to anchor yourself and feel strong and secure. You learned how to bring energies up from Mother Earth to cleanse yourself and help you feel supported.

Getting big in your energies is a good thing to do: You learned how to connect to a source of higher vibrational energy outside your body. You tuned in to the energies of healing, of unconditional love and light, and learned how to expand your energy field so that you can step into your true potential. You also learned how to send some of this energy to people you love.

You don't want to carry other people's energies: You've been doing clearing work throughout this book even though you might not have known what it's called. Breathing out anxiety is clearing it from your system. Like clearing the dye from the swimming pool, you've learned that raising your energies to a higher vibration clears out all the energies that are at a lower vibration. When you are at a high vibration and clear in your Life Force Energy, you are able to be your best self.

❖ ❖ ❖

When combined with conscious awareness, intention and permission, your Life Force Energy can be the key to creating stability and happiness in your life. It can help you feel more connected to your intuition, so you are aware of how you feel in your heart as well as what you think in your mind. A daily spiritual practice that keeps you connected to all of these aspects of your Self empowers you to be able to reach your full potential as a human being.

Clearing as a spiritual practice

Just as we can bring our energies back to ourselves, we can also send other people's energies back to them, gently and with love. Now in the case of Rosemary, it might not

benefit her to have her emotional pain come back, so we can also send it to Mother Earth to be processed, just as she processes our own anxieties and emotional pain.

Exercise: clearing your energy field

Here is a simple method for clearing other people's energies from your energy field. This is something that will really benefit you if you do it regularly, as part of your daily routine, as well as doing it when you feel you need to.

❖ Be centred in yourself, ground yourself, and know that you may be slightly 'off' because you're possibly carrying energies that don't belong to you.

❖ Set your intention out loud to clear (or in your mind if you're in a public place).

❖ Say the following: 'Any energies in my energy field that are not mine, I release to wherever they need to go, for the highest good of all.'

❖ Wait and see how you feel. You're stirring up your energy too, so you may actually be feeling residual emotions around the ones you've just released

❖ Feel your feet on the ground. Ground yourself more if you can.

We ask for the energies to be released for the highest good of all, because we don't really know what is best for others. For example, if Rosemary's friend was angry for being 'dumped on', she might try to send Rosemary back her own emotional pain. Perhaps that would make things significantly worse for Rosemary, and push her into

a clinical depression. We will never know all the answers. Rather than make the decision yourself, let the universe do what it does best.

Clearing around specific events or situations

Clearing other energies from our energy field isn't restricted to energies from people. When there is an event or a situation that involves many people, they might all invest their spiritual energies, including you, and it can get 'muddy' and difficult to focus when it comes to making a decision. An example might be a wedding, where too many people want to help with the arrangements, or a work situation where politics are involved.

Can you remember a situation or event that preoccupied you for a lot of time, weighing you down and making you feel drained just thinking of it? Did you feel like you wanted to run away? Sometimes feelings of avoidance are because your energy is being drained, and you don't have anything left to give. Your avoidance is not because you don't want to do it, or because you're being lazy, it's because you are scraping the bottom of the barrel when it comes to your energy levels, and you need to preserve yourself.

Exercise: clearing your energy field of a situation or group of people

This technique starts with you taking back the energies you've invested in the situation/event so you feel better in yourself. Then once you feel grounded and centred, you can give back the energies that are not yours. Use a situation from your past for this exercise now, so you can see how

it feels to release the energies around it. Then you can incorporate it into a spiritual practice and use it whenever you need to.

❖ Think of the situation in your mind, visualize it however you can, go back to the last time you were involved with it and recreate it in your imagination. Have it in freeze frame, as if you've stopped the video playing and everyone is standing still. Step into your body in this image, and allow yourself to feel what you were feeling in that moment. If it's too strong for you, you can turn down the intensity, a bit like turning down the volume on the stereo.

❖ Breathe and notice how you feel when you do this – notice the shift in your body as you take on the energies from that moment in time and space. Feel your feet on the ground.

❖ Imagine that your energy is like sparkly fairy dust (go on, try it!!) What colour is it? Visualize how it's distributed around the people in your mind, around the room.

❖ Ask for it to come back to you, clear and at a high vibration.

❖ Wait and imagine the sparkles gathering together, coming together into a ball of light. You're pulling your investment out of the situation.

❖ Let the ball of light enter your energy field. At this point, you may be feeling much calmer and more contained in yourself.

❖ Now breathe again, check in with your energy and sense if you have any energies that don't belong to you.

❖ Say the following: 'I give permission for any energies in my energy field that are not mine to leave now.'

❖ Wait again, breathe, soften, relax and let them leave. Notice how you feel.

Having the awareness that you may be carrying energies belonging to others or to situations enables you to disconnect from them and bring yourself back to yourself. Without the awareness, what usually happens is that we think it's all our own stuff and start to analyse what's going on, create negative thought patterns, get caught up in heavy emotions and make things worse.

If your first stop is always to clear your energies, and then check in and see how you feel, you get clearer on what is your stuff, and what is not. Using clearing techniques as part of a daily spiritual practice stops these energies from building up over time, and helps you have a better awareness and connection to yourself.

Taking back your energies as a daily spiritual practice

Sometimes we invest so much of ourselves in something that it might be difficult to call our energies back. We think about it all the time. We visualize what we want, we hope, dream, expect and get disappointed if it doesn't happen the way we want it to, when we want it to. We may feel we have some control over a situation or a person by being so invested, but in fact, our energies are jamming up the works.

The most amazing thing about using this technique is that when you take your energy back you free up space for the energies around whatever the issue is to clear by themselves. It's like the saying, 'If you love someone, set them free.' With a deep trust that everything *is* going to turn out in the best way possible, let go of your attachment to the outcome or a

need to control the situation. Take a step back, breathe and clear your energies and see what happens!

Exercise: retrieving energy

❖ Centre yourself in your body and check that you have permission from yourself to do this work. You might not have permission from your mind, so reach deep into your inner knowing and tell yourself you really don't have any control over this anyway. Let go of the worry around it first; if you can't control it, worrying won't help, releasing worry is like a cloud lifting, and sometimes you get clarity just by doing this.

❖ Breathe and calm and relax your body. If you are having trouble relaxing, you may want to do the grounding exercise.

❖ When you are ready, set your intention out loud: 'I take back my energy from (name the situation or person here). I release my need to control the situation or that person. I ask for my energies to come back now, cleansed and healed.'

❖ Wait, breathe and see how you feel. You might have had a flash in your mind, like a recognition or an answer to a question, or you might not; it doesn't matter.

❖ Breathe, ground and come back to centre.

❖ Do this again the next day, and the day after that, until you feel all your energy has come back completely.

How will you know when you've come back completely? When you feel more grounded and centred around the situation or person, when news of them doesn't throw

you off balance, when you don't feel as much emotional upheaval if you think about it.

What we think about, or worry about subconsciously, we 'feed' with our energy. So, when we set our conscious awareness to clear something, it's wonderful and it works, but then when we bring our focus to something else, our subconscious mind might slip back and reconnect to what we just disconnected from. This is why you have to do this work more than once. This is why you have to keep checking in even if it felt like you were fully disconnected from it.

Why does this happen? Well, these subconscious connections have probably taken some time to grow, and so it's not surprising that they may take some time to fade away. Keep going! There is usually work to be done on a deeper level. This is a process. You are learning a new way of using your energy as a resource for positive change and growth.

One way to help clear out negative thoughts and beliefs is to write them down and work through them. Write out a list of the things you are deeply worried about, and the negative thoughts you have about these situations, yourself, or anything else that is disturbing you. If you can clear them yourself with your energy work, then go for it! But don't be afraid to ask for help; remember that this work will help you free yourself up to have the happy life you deserve.

❖ ❖ ❖

Centring, grounding and expanding as a spiritual practice

Use the major exercises we have done for centring, grounding and expanding, and turn them into your own spiritual practice. Once you have put the time in, they get easier to do, and you can then do them over a shorter period of time.

For example, you could take five minutes to centre yourself, then take five minutes to ground yourself, then take another five minutes to expand. You might just want to take 10 minutes to ground, or another day you might prefer to take 15 minutes to expand.

Always notice how you feel and do only what you feel you need to do that day. Pushing yourself too hard is not healthy and may create a dislike in your subconscious mind of doing any energy work at all. You may also notice that as you are doing healing work, your mind concentrates on the work you are doing and lets go of thoughts that may upset you or worry you. Just that alone may be enough to help you feel more like yourself again.

This work is mindful. Bring your mind purposefully with you and away from worrying thoughts of the past and the future. Focus on something you are doing now, in the present moment.

❖ ❖ ❖

Mindfulness and Energy Healing as a spiritual practice

Anything you do mindfully can become a spiritual practice. You can wash the dishes and feel better afterwards, if while you're doing it you stop feeding your energies into anything that worries you. Just bring your focus of awareness into your centre, into your body and *experience*, and wash the dishes in a mindful way, instead of just doing it on autopilot.

To do this effectively, your thought process may be like this:

I run the tap, the water is warm. I get the sponge, I am pouring in the washing-up liquid, I mix the water and washing-up liquid and make bubbles. The bubbles are beautiful, the light touches off of them in a beautiful way. I put the plates and cutlery into the sink. I let them sit there and I look out of the window at the sky. The sun is going down, there are so many colours to see. The sky looks like a painting. I am breathing with the sky. I feel my feet on the ground, I can hear my breath. I bring my awareness back to the dishes and start to wash the first plate.

Not like this:

I run the tap, the water is warm. I get the sponge, I am pouring the washing-up liquid. I can see the price tag on the bottle and I remember going to the shop to buy it. My gosh, washing-up liquid is so expensive these days. This one was ridiculously expensive and that person on the till was so rude to me. I'm never going back into that shop again...

And certainly not like this (!):

> *I run the tap, the water is warm. I get the sponge, I am pouring in the washing-up liquid. I wonder how long this will take as I still need to complete that work project. Sigh. It should have been in last week. I really should have worked late last night to finish it, but I was too tired. I know that it will take at least another day or two before I can get it finished. I tried to tell my manager today but she was too busy to talk to me. I'm going to have to talk to her tomorrow about it; I hope they don't bring this up at my review meeting...*

Do you see what I mean? Staying in the present with what is happening now, in this moment, is a spiritual practice when you bring your full awareness into it. Feeding the present moment instead of what happened in the shop, or what is going on at work, is what fills your soul up. This is you, feeding yourself. This is mindfulness as an Energy Healing practice, giving you more energy for what life brings.

Exercise: mindful relaxation

Take about five minutes to do this exercise.

- ❖ Bring yourself into yourself by letting go of thoughts about anything other than what is happening now.

- ❖ Breathe and feel your feet on the ground, calm your mind and go into feeling.

- ❖ Feel your clothes on your body.

- ❖ Notice your hands. What do they look like?

❖ Turn them over and look at the lines on your hands. Follow them with your eyes.

❖ Do you feel your brain relaxing?

If you had trouble doing this, don't worry, it's a practice, and it takes practice!

Don't get angry or frustrated. Simply bring your focus and attention back to the present moment and start where you left off. You *will be* thinking thoughts. This is not about stopping thinking. It's about paying attention to what you are thinking so that you stay in the present moment. Remember, the more attention you feed to yourself, the less you feed the fears, then you end up with fewer fears and more of you.

It does get easier over time, so it stands to reason that when you start doing this, you will have more fears than you will once you get better at it. It's harder work in the beginning but so worthwhile.

What did you find your mind going back to most of the time? Is it a real fear or something that you are assuming is real? Get clear on it. You may want to write down everything that's on your mind connected to this fear, so you can get it all out into the open, and not hide from it. Remember, being authentic and true to yourself is part of Energy Healing too. Telling yourself that something is big and scary when it really isn't, takes you away from yourself and is an energy drain. And yes, talk to someone if you need to, take action if you need to.

If there is a real issue that is upsetting you, you will have to do something real about it.

❖ ❖ ❖

Fire up your daily practice with intention

By bringing your intention into mindfulness you can really connect to yourself. You can use power statements (affirmations) and clearing statements with mindfulness to create positive changes in your energy field.

In this next exercise the intention is to call all your energies back into your body. You can change the intention to be whatever you feel you need, such as receiving healing, becoming more relaxed or releasing emotional or physical pain.

Exercise: using intention and healing as spiritual practices

Take a few minutes to do this exercise. Bring your awareness and attention into the present moment.

❖ Start by voicing the main intention of the exercise, 'I call all my energy, from wherever I have invested it, to come back to my body now.'

❖ Wait and see how you feel. Breathe. If you need to centre yourself, do it. If you need to ground yourself, do it.

❖ Now move your focus of attention down (or up) your body, speaking (or thinking) your intention to each part of your physical body. For example:

– 'I bring my focus of awareness to my head.'

- 'I call all energies that are mine that belong in my head to come back now.'

- 'I bring my focus of awareness down to my face.'

- 'I call all energies from my face that may have left me, to come back now.'

❖ Work your way through your body, all the time staying in the present moment with your thoughts, all the time repeating the intention, so you might be saying things like 'I call all my energy that has left my head, to come back to my head,' and 'I call all my energy that has left my heart, to come back to my heart.' It's a bit like going in deeper and performing the healing on each body part, instead of doing it just for your body as a whole.

❖ When you've finished calling all your energy back, do spend some time drawing down the healing light and making sure the energies that have come back are cleansed and healed; you don't want them bringing back any emotional debris from wherever they may have come from!

You will find that by having a strong intention you automatically feel more contained in your physical body, you feel more centred and more grounded. There is a certainty and a focus when you have an intention, and using intention on a regular basis can increase your self-confidence and sense of self-worth too.

Other ideas for a mindful Energy Healing practice

You can bring mindfulness into anything – yoga, football, walking, even cleaning the house. Here are some ideas to start you off:

❖ Cook a mindful dinner, 'fill it' with healing energies and eat it mindfully. Notice how much better it tastes!

❖ Walk barefoot and feel the sensation of your feet touching the ground, the grass, the sand. Send healing into your feet, and send healing into the ground as you walk.

❖ Take a hot bath and connect to a healing energy of gratitude, washing every part of your body slowly, mindfully and with the healing energy of gratitude.

❖ Have a mindful cup of tea with yourself, centre yourself in your heart, connect to the healing light, infuse your tea with healing and as you sip, ask yourself if there is anything you need to know now, anything you are missing in your life. Have a notebook and pen beside you in case you want to write anything down.

The key is to be completely in the present moment, not to feed your energies into the past or the future. And as I said before, it will get easier, until you find your way of being is like this more of the time.

❖ ❖ ❖

Breathing as a spiritual practice

We have used breathing a lot in this book as a focus of our awareness, as an anchor to the present moment. We can use breathing to create a spiritual practice too. This is what we have done already with the breath:

❖ Using the breath to draw down the energy of uncon- ditional love, or to draw down the energy of healing.

❖ Using the breath to open up the flow in the body, to 'push' the energy of healing around our body.

❖ Using the breath to breathe out the lower, heavier vibrations of anxiety, fear, doubt, jealousy, anger, etc.

Here's a nice exercise. Use it every day for a week or so to see if it changes anything in your life.

Exercise: opening up to beauty

❖ Sit in a space of love. Bring the focus of your awareness into your body, connect into your centre, and then check that you are grounded.

❖ Imagine you are connecting the top of your head into a source of beauty. Wait until you feel you've connected in and notice how it feels: the texture, the brightness, the strength.

❖ Breathe in the beauty, and breathe out anything that is not beauty. Remember, the beauty you are breathing in is not you. It is an energetic source of beauty.

❖ Breathe in beauty, and feel your body opening up to beauty. Do you feel anxious doing this? Breathe out the anxiety. Go as deeply as you feel comfortable doing; each time you try this exercise you can go deeper.

❖ Breathe in Beauty. Breathe out all that is not beauty. Do this for five to 10 minutes, or longer if you want to.

❖ Let go of the breath and return to your natural breathing state.

❖ Ground, centre and close.

After doing this exercise with me in a session, one of my clients walked home and a complete stranger ran across the road to tell her that she was the most beautiful woman he had ever seen!

You can replace the energetic source of beauty with happiness, peace, joy, lightness, or gratitude. Choose something that you resonate with, stick with it for a few days and see how you feel.

❖ ❖ ❖

Who are you when you are your best, healed self?

There is always work to be done, even if you feel like you have reached enlightenment. Enlightened people still have to do the mundane day-to-day tasks like cleaning the house and doing the cooking! You will still have difficult days and wonderful days. The difference is you won't write off a whole day as a bad day if something upsets you, and you won't feel like a victim any more, needing something or someone to blame. If you need a rest, take a rest. Enlightened people get tired too!

One of my clients was visibly relieved when I told her that I make mistakes, that I have bad days and that I get upset by things just like she does. It's not that I see myself as enlightened, but I've been using Energy Healing as a daily spiritual practice for many years. I breathe it and live it all day, every day. The first thing I do before anything else is to clear my energies. Even in writing this book, I cleared all the energies in the way of it, so it could be the best book I could write in that moment! My point is this – I still get angry, I still get upset. The difference is, I process it quickly.

I let it go, rather than holding on to it for weeks and weeks and turning it into a grudge and never forgiving. I used to be like that – someone would say something nasty to me or behind my back, and I would be upset about it for months. It was like a wound that would never heal. Now it heals very much faster because I choose to focus on healing it, rather than letting it upset me.

Holding on to emotional pain makes your body sick and that brings with it physical pain. Doing your work, clearing the energies and expanding and healing yourself releases emotional pain, and opens up your body so that it can heal itself at the physical level. Looking after your thoughts prevents you from creating more emotional pain for yourself.

Become responsible for your energy!

These techniques are meant for you to use and to use frequently, as often as you need to. They have helped people move away from depression and be empowered. They have helped people feel more secure in their lives and 'grow out of' panic attacks and phobias. When you clear away other people's energies what's left is your own, and that's much easier to work with.

As you probably have figured out at this stage, underneath the moving flowing energies, deep in your subconscious, probably still lie limiting beliefs, fears and emotional pain that may not shift quickly and easily with Energy Healing alone. Do your healing work, and your energies will expand, your vibration will rise. It becomes easier to go deep and excavate the bigger pieces as you heal, so you truly begin

to resonate with all the good things you want in your life, and you start to see them coming in as a testimony to the work you are doing.

Once you're familiar with the techniques, do make the effort to use them in your daily life. Teach them to your friends, to your family, to your children. Play with them, have fun with them. Imagine a world where everyone is responsible for their own energy. That's a world I want to live in!

Resources

In this resource section I cover asking for help, books to read and how I can help you.

Asking for help

This section is by no means complete. Throughout the book, I have said 'Don't be afraid to ask for help,' so I wanted to give you some understanding of what type of help there is. In my years of experience as a therapist, I have found that clients feel disempowered at times by therapists. My aim here is to give you information that will empower you to ask good questions before you make a booking, and to know your rights when it comes to therapy, so that you can make the right decision for yourself based on your own good judgement and intuition.

Many people decide to train in a specific therapy and become a therapist instead of actually going into process as a client. If you do want to become a therapist, you will become a stronger, more authentic therapist if you begin as a client and make a good start on your own work before beginning any training programmes. You will also gain the

knowledge of what it is like to be a client, which enhances your personal skills if you decide to become a therapist!

Choosing a therapy

There are so many types of therapies to choose from it can be very confusing. I've listed and categorized some of the therapies here to make it a bit easier. I have not included **all** the different types of therapies that exist, just the more common ones. My descriptions are not definitive; they are brief, to give you a taste of what the therapy is about. If something appeals to you, I do urge you to look further into it to help you make up your mind.

Counselling: talking with someone to help you gain perspective on your life situation, this is non-directive, no advice is given and it is driven by the client i.e. the client chooses what to talk about. Counselling usually takes about four to six sessions to work through an issue.

Psychotherapy: this can be more directive, in that once it is clear what the client is looking to do, the therapist takes a more active role; they can suggest techniques and a direction to work in, using different processes to help create transformation. There may be homework in the form of tasks to do (such as keeping a journal), so for this reason several sessions may be required.

Psychoanalysis: very intensive, where the psychoanalyst studies your thought patterns and history and makes a diagnosis over many sessions. You do most of the talking, the therapist asks questions and traditionally sits behind you, out of eye contact. This may involve going back to trauma and childhood events, talking about dreams, etc.

Bereavement Counselling: a specialized form of counselling that helps you move on from a loss in your life – any kind of loss, not just the loss of a loved one.

Cognitive Behavioural Therapy: this psychotherapeutic process concentrates on looking at your thought patterns and teaching you ways to change them to more healthy ones.

Gestalt: a process that uses talking and feeling to work through problems. This type of therapy works on a holistic approach, working with the emotional body; it can be very powerful and at times it may feel like the mindfulness Energy Healing exercises.

Human Givens: a type of psychotherapy that works on a framework based on the idea that people have a set of needs that have to be met.

Transpersonal Therapy: psychotherapy that works with a belief in God or something greater than us to help manage life situations.

Other forms of therapy may include: positive psychology, art therapy, brief therapy, family therapy, group therapy, play therapy, transactional therapy. You can see there are many different forms!

Therapy is really more about the relationship you create with the therapist than the type of therapy they are offering. So you do need to make an emotional connection with your therapist. Many psychotherapists use an integrative approach, which means that they are versed in several different modes of therapy and they blend them together as

needed in a session. The number of sessions that are required for psychotherapy/counselling are set between you and the therapist, and it can be decided up-front or on a session-by-session basis. However, if you feel you are not enjoying the process, are not connecting with, or not comfortable with the therapist, you can end the sessions at any time.

It's very useful to talk about the therapy process with the therapist i.e. check in and tell the therapist you're really benefitting from the sessions, or let them know if you're not happy. Talking about the therapy process with the therapist can dramatically improve the results as both of you are more aware of what is going on. Remember, sometimes it can be your resistance to the work making you unhappy with therapy, rather than anything the therapist is doing.

Keep in mind that a one-to-one session may be what you need if you're feeling fragile. Group therapy is when a group of people go into process together, and not always at the same time. This means that you will become exposed to other people's processes. If you pick up on their energies as well as the ones you are already trying to work with, it can really make things more difficult for you if you're not ready for it.

Questions to ask a psychotherapist/counsellor
1. How long have you been in practice?

2. Are you a member of an accrediting body? / Do you have a licence?

3. Where did you get your degree?

4. How much do you charge for your sessions?

5. Do I need to sign up for a certain number of sessions?

6. Do you have a cancellation policy?

7. Do you accept personal health insurance?

Energy therapies

When receiving Energy Healing there is no need for you to remove your clothing. You will typically lie down and the therapist will place their hands on or over your body, drawing down the Universal Life Force Energy into your biofield. These therapies can work over plaster casts if you have a broken limb, they can also work over distance if you cannot make it into the therapist's office for a treatment.

Types of energy therapies include:

❖ Bioenergy healing

❖ Crystal healing

❖ EmoTrance

❖ Hands of light holistic healing

❖ Integrated energy therapy (IET)

❖ Johrei

❖ Life alignment therapy

❖ Past life regression

❖ Pranic healing

❖ Quantum touch

❖ Rahinni

❖ Reconnection healing

- ❖ Reiki (there are many forms – Usui, Karuna, Tibetan, Angelic, Tera Mai, Rainbow, Dragon, Kundalini – all of which have different methods to access the Universal Life Force Energy)

- ❖ Restorative touch

- ❖ Sakara

- ❖ Seichem

- ❖ ThetaHealing®

You can research each type of healing, if you wish to know more about it. I would also suggest that you look for a recommendation from someone who has been to the healer before. Remember, this is more about the healer than about the modality of healing; some people are born to be healers and may not even have trained formally, so they may simply offer you 'spiritual healing'. Others who have trained for years may not be natural healers but may do a great job helping you release energies and acting as a witness for you. You will only know if you try it.

Many therapists tend to mix several therapies together and don't usually tell the client in advance, so ask when booking if it's pure Reiki, for example, or if they combine it with something else.

Remember everyone is different, and the training is different too. Each Reiki Master Teacher will teach in their own way, so Reiki students will all receive a different training. When looking for a therapist do your homework first – look at their website, read their blog, get a feel for their energy. Nowadays, there is online training available for Energy

Healers, and you can complete the masters' programme over a very short period of time. This **does not** make you a master therapist. However, some people call themselves that regardless. You need to be sure that you are going to a well-practiced professional. It's useful to ask some, or all, of the following questions.

Questions to ask an energy therapist

1. How long have you been providing Energy Healing treatments?

2. How much do you charge for a session?

3. What level of training do you have?

4. Where did you train? / Was your training in person with a teacher in a hands-on setting, or online?

5. When did you complete your training?

6. How many client hours have you completed?

7. Have you got full public liability insurance?

8. Can I contact one of your clients for a reference?

9. What should I expect in a session?

10. Do you practise healing on yourself every day?

If the therapist gets worried or angry with you for asking these questions, they might not be the right person for you. The last question, about self-healing and self-care, is **very important** – as a therapist, they will be seeing many people, and if they do not look after themselves, clear and raise their own vibrations, they may be passing their clients' energy over to you, and you don't want that.

Psychic readings are not part of an Energy Healing session. After the session, if the therapist has information for you based on what they read in your energies, treat it as information that is true for that therapist, in that moment.

Nothing has to be set in stone. Everything can change. Sometimes additional information from a therapist is useful, such as 'You are not really grounded in your body, perhaps you should spend some time doing that for yourself, and you'll feel better.' Do not deeply embrace everything you hear; only pay attention to it if it resonates with you. As you do your work, you get clearer on what your work is, and will be more empowered to decide yourself what you need to do.

Therapies that combine both talking and Energy Healing

The following therapies combine talking with energetic healing:

❖ **Emotional Freedom Technique (EFT):** uses tapping on energy points and affirmations in a set framework to shift energy and work with thought patterns.

❖ **Shamanism:** Shamanic methods vary dramatically depending on the training and background of the practitioner. You really need to investigate the therapist before you book a Shamanic healing session, do find out where they trained and how long they have been in practice. Consider getting a recommendation before booking, as this therapy really does depend on the individual practitioner.

❖ **Hypnotherapy:** the therapist goes into your subconscious mind and inserts a script or a programme to change a behaviour, or transform an irrational fear. It can involve energy work or not, depending on the therapist.

❖ **Energy Coaching:** there are many coaches out there offering energy work; be clear, however, that coaching is not always therapeutic. (Imagine a coach on a running field shouting at an athlete!) Coaching can help you set goals and get more confident, while therapy is something that I believe should be loving, gentle and transformational.

Therapies that work with the body

Even though they are focused directly on the physical body, bodywork therapies can really help release blocked emotions and are a great complement to any energy work or psychotherapeutic work you may be doing.

❖ **Massage:** there are many different types of massage depending on how deep and strong a treatment you wish to receive.

❖ **Shiatsu:** a type of massage where the therapist can release trapped energies from the muscles, as well as working with the physical muscles in the body.

❖ **Reflexology:** using pressure points on the feet to heal the whole body energetically.

❖ **Reiki massage:** the therapist combines Reiki with physical massage.

❖ **Rolfing:** releasing energies within the connecting fibres and tissues in the body.

The questions to ask before booking a bodywork treatment are similar to the ones already listed above.

Combining bodywork with Energy Healing

You can incorporate Energy Healing into body movements to create a strong, grounding practice that will keep you healthy. Healing may not always be the intention behind the class, but sometimes you will find it 'sneaks' its own way in. Make sure the facilitator is experienced, and you feel safe within the group. Try a drop-in class before you sign up for a whole term. This type of practice would be more about maintenance of a good energetic state, rather than a portal into doing deep transformational work. However, people have been known to experience deep healing during this type of work, even though it's not necessarily the intention behind the class.

❖ Biodanza

❖ Chakra dancing

❖ Qigong

❖ Seven rhythms dancing

❖ Tai chi

❖ Yoga: there are many traditional forms of Yoga such as Hatha, Astanga, Kundalini, Raja, etc., and many new non-traditional forms such as Bikram, Iyengar, Anti-Gravity and Laughter, to name a few.

Therapies for the environment

You might find after doing energy work that you want to change the energies in your house, or in your place of work.

❖ **Feng shui:** the practitioner will come and survey your building and give recommendations around where to put particular types of furniture, what colours to use and how to position items for the optimum energy flow.

❖ **House/Land Clearing:** there are land healers who are Shamans, they can come to your house/workplace and work directly with energy blocks in the land. If the energy is being disrupted by a power line, they can help you work around it to improve the general energy flow in the space.

Further reading

You can heal yourself and then harness the power of the energy around you to create the life you've always wanted. Don't take my word for it, go read what these other people say and try it for yourself! These are some of my favourite books that have helped me on my own healing journey. There are lots more out there too, so choose something that resonates with you.

E-Squared, Pam Grout (Hay House, 2013)
Nine energy experiments that you can use to work with the Universal Life Force Energy for manifestation.

Frequency, Penny Peirce (Beyond Words/Atria, Simon & Schuster 2009)
Getting bearings on your personal energy frequency and how to raise your vibration.

The Game of Life and How to Play It, Florence Scovel-Shinn (Waiting in the Other Room Productions, 2014)
The original book on manifestation and energy.

The Heart's Note, Stewart Pearce (Findhorn Press, 2010)
There are some wonderful practical exercises in here to help you open your heart and connect more deeply to the vibration of your soul.

The Lightworker's Way, Doreen Virtue (Hay House, 2005)
A wonderful story about what it means to discover you are a healer and how it can impact your life.

Power vs Force, David R. Hawkins MD, PhD (Hay House, 2014)
This book is a wonderful explanation of the vibrations of different emotional energies.

A Return to Love, Marianne Williamson (Thorsons, 1996)
The story of Marianne's journey of healing, interspersed with the philosophy of *A Course in Miracles.*

Shaman, Healer, Sage, Alberto Villoldo (Bantam, 2001)
Full of ways to work with energy, as well as a different perspective on life.

Soul Retrieval, Sandra Ingerman (HarperOne, 2010)
A remarkable book about our Life Force Energy and the Shamanic technique of Soul Retrieval.

You Can Heal Your Life, Louise Hay (Hay House, 2004)
Reviews the different parts of the body and what it means when there is illness, dis-ease or blocks in them.

Why People Don't Heal and How They Can, Caroline Myss (Bantam, 1998)
This book may help explain any resistance you may be having to the healing process. Lots to think about here.

Zero Limits, Joe Vitale (John Wiley & Sons, 2009)
How energy clearing can transform your life and change the world.

How I can help you

I have some free resources that you can claim right away as a reader of this book, so do come and have a look. My mission is 'to heal the world by teaching people how to heal themselves,' and to that end my website has many resources to help further your Energy Healing journey. Visit www.abby-wynne.com for more information.

My other books

Energy Healing for Everyone: A Practical Guide to Self-Healing (Balboa Press, 2012)
Exercises and practical ideas to help you bring Energy Healing into your life.

Spiritual Tips for Enlightenment: Practical Spirituality for Every Week of the Year (CreateSpace Independent Publishing Platform, 2013)
Practical ways to bring spirituality into your life.

Healing meditations

I have recorded several healing meditations and healing sessions to help you as you work. Some of them are similar to the exercises included in this book, and they may enable

you to work through blocks and help you to reach a deeper level. Let my voice guide you through the session, and you can experience healing wherever and whenever you feel you need extra support.

I also offer online classes, one-to-one Skype sessions and a healing circle, which you can join and then receive Energy Healing from me twice a month. Visit www.abby-wynne.com for more information.

ABOUT THE AUTHOR

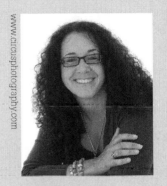

Abby Wynne is a Shamanic Psychotherapist and Energy Healer working in private practice. She teaches people how to reconnect to their hearts and become empowered in their healing process. She has four beautiful children and lives with her family in Dublin, Ireland.

For information about how to work with Abby, or for her other books, worksheets and recorded meditations, visit her website

www.abby-wynne.com

Notes

Notes

Notes

Notes

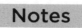
Notes

HAY HOUSE BASICS
Online courses

If you're interested in finding out more about the topics that matter most for improving your life, why not take a Hay House Basics online course?

Each course is intended to provide a powerful introduction to a core topic in the area of self-development or mind, body, spirit. Presented by a renowned expert, each course includes:

An overview of the topic, including its application and benefits

•

Video demonstrations of practical exercises

•

Meditations and visualizations to guide you

•

Specially created text guides, available to download for future reference

Available at a special low price, these courses are the ultimate route to a full spiritual life!

Find out more at **www.hayhousebasics.com**

Made in the USA
San Bernardino, CA
08 March 2018